The Art of Getting Well

DEDICATION

To June, to Darcy, to Aisha, and to everyone who helped make this book a reality. And if you wonder if you might possibly belong on this list, believe me, you do. Thank you.

Ordering

Trade bookstores in the U.S. and Canada please contact:

Publishers Group West
1700 Fourth Street, Berkeley CA 94710
Phone: (800) 788-3123   Fax: (800) 351-5073

Hunter House books are available at bulk discounts for textbook course adoptions; to qualifying community, health-care, and government organizations; and for special promotions and fund-raising. For details please contact:

Special Sales Department
Hunter House Inc., PO Box 2914, Alameda CA 94501-0914
Phone: (510) 865-5282   Fax: (510) 865-4295
E-mail: ordering@hunterhouse.com

Individuals can order our books from most bookstores, by calling **(800) 266-5592**, or from our website at **www.hunterhouse.com**

The Art of
GETTING
WELL

A Five-Step Plan for Maximizing Health
When You Have a Chronic Illness

DAVID SPERO, R.N., BSN

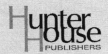

Hunter House Inc., Publishers
PO Box 2914
Alameda CA 94501-0914

Library of Congress Cataloging-in-Publication Data

Spero, David.
The art of getting well : a five-step plan for maximizing health when you have a
chronic illness / David Spero ; foreword by Martin Rossman.—1st ed.
p. cm.
Includes bibliographical references.
ISBN-13: 978-0-89793-357-5 (cloth)—ISBN-13: 978-0-89793-356-8 (paper)
ISBN-10: 0-89793-357-5 (cloth)—ISBN-10: 0-89793-356-7 (paper)
1. Chronic diseases—Alternative treatment. 2. Health. 3. Holistic medicine. 4. Self-care,
Health. I. Title.
RC108 .S66 2001
615.5—dc21   2001039722

Project Credits

Cover Design: Peri Poloni, Knockout Design   Book Design and Production: Jinni Fontana
Copy Editor: Kelley Blewster   Proofreader: John David Marion
Acquisitions Editor: Jeanne Brondino   Editorial and Production Assistant: Emily Tryer
Associate Editor: Alexandra Mummery   Publicity Manager: Sara Long
Sales and Marketing Assistant: Earlita K. Chenault   Order Fulfillment: Lakdhon Lama
Customer Service Manager: Christina Sverdrup   Computer Support: Peter Eichelberger
Administrator: Theresa Nelson   Publisher: Kiran S. Rana

Manufactured in the United States of America

9 8 7 6 5 4   First Edition   08 09 10 11 12

CONTENTS

FOREWORD

There are several things you need to know about my friend and colleague David Spero, the author of this wonderful book.

First, he's "been there" in person. He's been a patient and a person living with multiple sclerosis for over twelve years, and he walks his talk, living fully, even thriving with it, in spite of it, and partially because of the way he's responded to it.

Second, he knows what he's talking about on a professional level. David is a registered nurse and a health coach who has specialized for many years in working with people living with chronic illnesses. He's developed curricula for self-care courses, for public health programs, and for scores of individuals from many walks of life with many different health challenges.

Third, he's a really fine writer. I have a confession to make. After thirty years of practicing, researching, writing, speaking, and teaching in the field of holistic medicine, I remain as passionate about the topic as ever—*but* I am sick of reading books about self-healing. They are generally so repetitive and preachy I can barely stand to look at them. By contrast, I read this book through in one sitting and was left wanting to hear more. David has a gift of making things simple yet interesting, of passing along useful information in a brief, pointed, and often funny way. Once you read the opening chapter title, "Studies Show Life Is Hard," you know you are in the hands of someone who knows what he's talking about.

Finally, David is a kind and generous man who has dedicated himself to helping others. David always signs his e-mails with the phrase "Your friend, David," and he acts that way in all of his interactions.

David's health-coaching motto is "Illness is the best teacher, awareness is the best medicine, self-care is the best care." He aims to show us the truth and wisdom of that statement, and he succeeds in the pages that follow.

I am honored to be able to write a foreword for such a book. I commend you to the good hands of David Spero—our friend in the business of getting ourselves well.

— Martin L. Rossman, M.D., Dipl. Ac. (N.C.C.A.O.M.)

Important Note

The material in this book is intended to provide a review of maximizing health and well-being when you have a chronic illness. Every effort has been made to provide accurate and dependable information. However, you should be aware that professionals in the field may have differing opinions, and change is always taking place. If any of the treatments described herein are used, they should be undertaken only under the guidance of a licensed health-care practitioner. The author, editors, and publishers cannot be held responsible for any error, omission, professional disagreement, outdated material, or adverse outcomes that derive from use of any of these treatments in a program of self-care or under the care of a licensed practitioner.

PREFACE

I wrote *The Art of Getting Well* for two of my favorite kinds of people. First are those, like me, who live with conditions labeled "chronic" or "progressive," who have been told we can't get better, we must get worse, and there's not much we can do about it. Second are people, like me, who get paid as health professionals to help the first group, often botching the job. The book has wider applications, though. Since chronic conditions are so varied, and the issues each brings up are so similar, anyone interested in health and wellness will probably enjoy and benefit from this book.

The Art of Getting Well owes much to the Chronic Disease Self-Management Program, run by Kate Lorig at Stanford University. Leading CDSMP groups taught me that no matter how difficult our lives, how blocked and defeated we seem, there is always a way forward. In these groups, we all help each other, regardless of diagnosis. The experience of a person with one illness will frequently illuminate a path for people with another.

The art of getting well is a martial art, a gentle form of self-defense. Like a martial art, it emphasizes awareness and balance. Our genetic inheritance, our exposure to harmful environments, our social and economic conditions, our problems with work and relationships, the habits we picked up before we knew better—these are not our fault, but they can damage us. And it is our responsibility to minimize the damage and maximize our well-being. When life makes us sick, we can fight back with self-care. We can change the conditions that injure us and adapt to the things we cannot change. This book provides a host of skills to help you develop your art, concentrating most of them into five steps: slowing down, getting help, making change, valuing your body and your life, and self-managing your condition.

This book is not always positive. That would be ridiculous, given the subject matter. Acknowledging the anger, fear, and grief that often accompany major illness, *The Art of Getting Well* shows how we can use such painful feelings to change harmful situations, motivate healthier behaviors, and learn compassion for ourselves.

In spite of the heavy subject matter, *The Art of Getting Well* aims to be consistently entertaining and inspirational. Some of it is actually fun. You'll hear great stories, meet amazing people, and discover remarkable science, and you'll ground this inspiration in specific, practical steps you can take to start getting well.

What makes *The Art of Getting Well* different from other health books? First, it demonstrates that we can get better—not just slow the progression of illness, not just cope, but improve—no matter how we're labeled, how long we've been sick, or how many therapies we've tried. Whether it's heart disease, arthritis, lupus, depression, fibromyalgia, or any other "chronic" diagnosis, we can often stabilize our disease process and improve our overall condition. Second, this book maintains that we get better not through willpower and following orders but by improving the quality of our lives, a view backed by scientific research but ignored by most clinicians. As we master the art of getting well, we can often achieve better, more fulfilling lives than we had before our illness.

Most important, this book recognizes that the key to improving our quality of life, and thus our health, lies in overcoming barriers to self-care. Most of us would take better care of ourselves if we could, but formidable practical, psychological, and spiritual obstacles can block our way. *The Art of Getting Well* identifies those barriers and gives practical solutions for overcoming them.

☞ To My Health-Care Colleagues

This book is for you, as much as for my friends with chronic conditions. (Let's face it: we're frequently the same people.) *The Art of Getting Well* will help you understand and deal with those of us who have difficulty with self-care, your much beloved "noncompliant" patients.

The book is based on science; the studies and references are listed at the back. Fascinating as the science is, though, it's not what the book is about. It's about learning to take care of ourselves, finding reasons to do so, and overcoming the barriers in our way. Most doctors, nurses, and therapists I have known could use this knowledge in their own lives.

I came by the wisdom in this book honestly. In twenty-seven years of nursing, I have coached and cared for hundreds of people with a wide variety of chronic conditions. Twelve years ago I became one of them, when I was diagnosed with multiple sclerosis. Since then, I have researched scores of books and hundreds of studies and interviewed dozens of people with different diagnoses. I have pursued a series of self-care avenues, paying careful attention to the results, and studied with some great healers and teachers.

I owe a debt to Dr. Martin Rossman and the Academy for Guided Imagery (AGI). More than any other process, imagery helped me with my own illness, and my training in guided imagery taught me just how tightly body and mind are linked. AGI also taught me much about psychology, especially cognitive-behavioral therapy, the third guiding light of my practice and this book.

Most of all, I am grateful to the hundreds of people I have interviewed, nursed, and coached. I have learned more from them than from anyone else, not just about health, but about life. I am glad, honored, and proud to be able to share their knowledge with you.

— DAVID SPERO, R.N.

STUDIES SHOW LIFE IS HARD

One thing I learned early. Being a victim just doesn't work.

AIDS survivor Rob Mitchell

THIS BOOK IS ABOUT GETTING WELL when life seems weighted against the possibility of our doing so. It explains how we can recover our health and improve our lives, despite "chronic" problems for which medicine has no cure. In these pages you will find all the ideas and inspiration you need for successful self-care; you will read about ways to get better even in difficult circumstances.

Here's an example of what we're up against, and how self-care helps. When Cindy Wong was forty-five, she already had hypertension, thyroid disease, and clinical depression. "I wasn't taking care of myself," she remembers, which is understandable, since her husband had left her, with a rebellious daughter, aging parents, and a stressful job. "I didn't complain," she says. "In our culture, you're not supposed to."

Then she found herself in the emergency room, bleeding heavily from what turned out to be uterine cancer. Facing yet another illness, Cindy got fed up. She recalls:

Lying there, waiting for surgery, I promised, "If I make it through this, I am going to start doing something for myself." I couldn't have told you what that meant but I'd been taking care of everyone but me, and that had to change. Afterward, I went to the hospital's health-education office to see what they offered. I signed up for stress-reduction programs and stretching classes. Later, I started exercising and meditating.

It took me years to realize I had to put myself first. I cut back work to four days a week. I still take care of my parents, I'm still there for my daughter, but I make sure I get to my programs and do my meditation every day. My self-esteem is higher, because I'm taking time out for myself. My family relationships are actually better than ever; I have more energy, and my health has been improving.

Cindy isn't out of the woods yet, and she will probably never be able to throw away her medicines or party like a teenager. But she has taken control of her life, stabilized her condition, improved her general health, and become a positive, lively person, a joy to be around—no small accomplishment for a woman in her situation. Getting well or overcoming illness doesn't necessarily mean cure, and it doesn't mean living forever. Nor does it mean a list of dos and don'ts, pills to take, and foods to avoid. It means improving our condition and gradually making our lives happier, healthier, more fulfilling. How much our health improves depends on the severity of our illness, the conditions of our lives, and the internal and external resources we can bring to bear. How much better we feel depends mostly on us.

☙ So What's New About This?

Unlike some other self-care books, this one doesn't say we make ourselves sick or think ourselves well. It doesn't say, "Take control of your life," while glossing over the difficulties involved. It doesn't even say, "Follow your doctor's orders." Instead, it gives a practical, five-step program for recovery:

1. **Slow down.** Save some energy for your body and life, instead of giving every last ounce to work, worry, other demands, or entertainment.

2. **Make a change.** Change something in your life that is damaging. No matter how small, any successful change builds self-confidence and makes the next change easier.

3. **Get help.** None of us can do it alone; life is a cooperative effort. Learn to find and ask for help.

4. **Value your body and your life.** Listen to your body and treat it with respect. Fill your life with more pleasure, love, and reasons to live.

5. **Grow up.** Educate yourself, take responsibility, be assertive. Accept yourself the way you are, but don't give up on getting better.

These steps would sound intimidating, even to me, except for three things. First, we rarely need the whole program. Anything we do for ourselves is likely to pay dividends. Second, every single step should feel good; the whole idea, supported by scientific studies, is that improving quality of life will improve our health. Third, you're probably doing many things right already.

So it's not as hard as it sounds. In these pages, we will meet people who have carried out this program, over years, one step at a time. They have overcome AIDS, heart disease, arthritis, chronic fatigue, lupus, fibromyalgia, asthma, cancer, and other conditions, including, in my case, multiple sclerosis. These are people I have nursed, interviewed, or coached, not an elite group, but people with problems like those we all have. If they can do it, you can, too.

I am not promising any picnic or any miracles, though picnics are good for you, and miracles happen all the time. Overcoming chronic conditions is a challenge; it calls for all our intelligence, courage, and creativity and all the help we can get. Barriers will block our way, and sometimes we won't even know they're there, just that we're stuck. This book will help identify and overcome them. With effort, time, and a few breaks, we may find the journey of recovery leading us to better lives and better health than we had ever thought possible.

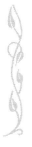

ᴂ Not Our Fault

Before planning how to get well, it may help to consider the various reasons we get sick, only a few of which are under our control. Sometimes our genes are programmed for susceptibility to one or another awful disease. Some environments subject us to toxic chemicals, natural or man-made, while others are full of hostile organisms. Some of us live amid violence, without ever knowing physical safety, or in crazy families who deprive us of emotional security and self-respect. We may lack sufficiently healthy food or water. We may grow up without opportunities for exercise, fresh air, education, relaxation, or love.

Studies of stressful life events—job loss, divorce, relocation, death of a family member, etc.—consistently show higher rates of all types of disease following such stressors. To these, we can add all of our maladaptive responses to life's insults: bad posture, attitudes, or diets, unacknowledged emotions, lack of exercise, overwork, hurry, various forms of self-abuse and addiction. All of these injurious behaviors were learned somewhere or adopted before we knew better, for reasons that were necessary—or at least seemed like good ideas—at the time.

Most diseases, then, except for overwhelming infections or pure genetic defects, arise from numbers of factors stretching back through our lives and heredity and outward through all our social and environmental influences, a web of causation that we can never completely sort out. For various reasons, our bodies (and minds) do not get their needs met, and they react by getting sick. Our bodies weren't made to last forever, and years of wear and tear eventually cause breakdowns.

Therefore, it makes no sense to blame ourselves for illness, to feel guilty about things we could not control. Guilt doesn't do anyone any good. Far worse than guilt, though, is helplessness, the feeling that turns us into victims without hope of salvation. Research shows that people with high "self-efficacy" (the belief that we can do the things we set out to do) and "internal locus of control" (the belief that we control much of what happens to us) have fewer complications, less distress, and slower progression of illness than those who feel less powerful. Although we often don't know how much, if any, influence we actually have, we're better off acting as though we do have influence. As we'll see in Chapter 6, we often have more control than we realize.

Fight Back with Self-Care

Though it's not a universal reaction, we have a right to grieve, to be angry, and often to be a little scared about health problems. The question is, what do we do with those feelings? This book says that when life makes us sick, we can fight back with self-care. Use anger as motivation to change harmful life situations (like a stressful job or a family that continues to smoke despite our lung disease). Employ fear of future complications as a reason to change unhealthy behaviors and attitudes. Allow sadness to extend into feelings of compassion, and even love, for our bodies and our whole selves, who struggle with so much difficulty.

Chronic conditions are not our fault, but no one else will fix them for us, nor can they. Only we can take care of ourselves. We can't change our genes or our age, but everything else is up for grabs. We can even delay or modify the expression of our bad genes in many cases.

The same dynamic applies whether we have arthritis, herpes, hepatitis, depression, or any other health problem. The disease is there; it has genetic, historical, or environmental causes. Our response to it, though, makes a huge difference in how much we suffer and how likely we are to get well. Even for conditions labeled "chronic" or "progressive," we can often slow, stop, or reverse the rate of progression or recurrence and the severity of symptoms by employing measures such as the ones described in this book.

Health Reflects Life

Annoying fact: The better our lives, the better our health is likely to be. Studies show that life is unfair in this way. Among these findings: Low job satisfaction is the number-one predictor for future heart attacks. Socio-economic standing—income, educational level, and power—predicts general health better than any other single factor except age.

It gets worse. College students who remembered loving relationships with their parents have been found, thirty years later, to have far less illness than those whose parental relationships were more strained. People who believe their spouses love them live longer. People with more friends are healthier. Laughter and happiness make the immune system work better. Sex is good for you; fun is good for you. People who report lower stress levels have lower blood pressures and stronger hearts.

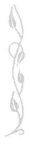

It is almost as if our bodies know how we feel about our lives, as if our immune systems and all our other miraculous self-healing mechanisms get discouraged when we get discouraged, as if they feel hopelessness, grief, and stress when we feel these ways. It's not just that happy people exercise more or eat better—though they tend to. "Mind/body" research demonstrates that our bodies, especially our unconscious self-care systems (such as the immune system), react to our life situations as strongly as do our conscious selves.

The immune system's sensitivity to life conditions has been proven beyond reasonable doubt. A 1977 Australian study, often replicated, found that T-lymphocytes (a type of white blood cell) were less active in people whose spouses had recently died. When researchers isolated the lymphocytes and put them in a test tube with a protein they would normally attack, the "bereaved" cells made only a halfhearted attempt to fight. It was like the cells were saying, "What's the use? Without my beloved, it's just not worth it." Of course, blood cells do not "think" in this sense, but the result is the same. The wounds of recently bereaved people also heal more slowly than those of others. In a number of studies, students with fewer friends, or more stress, have shown decreased immune responses in comparison to their peers.

Studies of heart patients have found that severity of blocked arteries and frequency of heart attacks vary greatly with a number of life situations, including quality of marriage, satisfaction at work, number of friends, even owning a good dog. I am certain that other body systems will be found responsive to life conditions, as soon as someone looks. If nothing else, every organ from the skin to the bowels reacts negatively to too much stress.

Science is telling us that we cannot separate our health from our lives. Stress, loss, isolation, economic insecurity, and other hardships tend to make us sick. Self-confidence, love, happiness, and relaxation are examples of conditions that help us heal. Therefore, getting well is largely a question of improving our quality of life.

~ My Ticket Out of Here

Sometimes sickness is a logical answer to life's pressures, a syndrome I call "illness is my one and only ticket out of here." When demands become overwhelming, when our lives become too tense, too stressful, too painful or crazy, and when we lack the ability or willingness to change them, our bodies may escape by getting sick, or even dying.

We can see this in some children diagnosed with "failure to thrive." Kids who are neglected or abused sometimes stop growing. Their glands simply stop producing growth hormones. Often, when these children go to hospitals or foster homes, the hormones kick in, and they start growing again. But when they are sent back to the place where they've been neglected, even if they get adequate food and shelter, they may once again shut down their growth processes. Obviously, this is not done consciously; it is the body's response to intolerable conditions.

Similar things happen to adults. My former nurse manager, Margaret Washington, had terribly high blood pressure, what doctors call "malignant hypertension." She took three medicines and still frequently ran numbers like 230/120, which would justify an emergency room visit for you or me. At fifty-five years old, she was somewhat overweight and under-exercised, but not nearly enough to account for her life-threatening pressure readings.

Margaret had worked her way up from the bottom, all the way from a nurse's aide to a manager with a master's degree, while raising children and, later, grandchildren. In spite of her accomplishments, she never felt respected or safe among our administration. As virtually the only African American in nursing leadership, she felt scrutinized and judged. Whether or not this feeling was accurate, it left her constantly anxious. She tried to work harder than everyone else, worried all the time, and took great pains not to offend or upset anyone in management. Because of her family's financial needs, she was unwilling to resign. She was on her way to a stroke, heart attack, or kidney failure, and it looked like a short trip.

What saved Margaret was a twisted blessing. To cut expenses, the company offered her a decent retirement package, and she grabbed it. Within four days, her blood pressure was on its way down. It continued dropping for the next three months, and currently she is on only one medication and has a normal blood pressure. She took a part-time job teaching parenting skills to young single mothers, which she had long wanted to do.

Was the job making Margaret sick, was it her genes, or was she making herself sick? I would call it a combination, but one thing is clear: If she

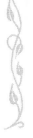

hadn't gotten out of there when she did, she likely would have gotten out crippled, or in a coffin.

☞ The Activity/Pain Cycle

Margaret was living the fatal version of what chronic-pain specialists call the activity/pain cycle. People with chronic pain often work and push themselves until pain makes them stop. Then they'll rest for the minimum possible time and try to resume working until pain stops them again.

When I heard about the activity/pain cycle, I thought, "This doesn't apply just to pain; it applies to every symptom and illness." Illness protects us by allowing us to stop beating our head against the wall, allowing us to take a break from endless demands and stress. Since our bodies desperately need us to stop, we aren't likely to get well unless we find some way to protect ourselves. Illness can often be seen as the body screaming for help.

One treatment goal in chronic pain is to move people to an activity/ rest cycle, where the person follows his or her body's rhythms and stops activity before pain builds up. Following the activity/rest cycle, people wind up doing more and suffering less. However, most find it very hard to make this particular change. Our society essentially lives a mass version of the activity/pain cycle, where it's not okay to stop until we break down. It's not okay to ask for help until we are disabled, and it's not okay to take a day off without a doctor's certificate.

Doctors have a term for taking advantage of illness to get some relief from the struggles of life; they call it "secondary gain." These gains can include more rest, attention from family and health-care providers, sympathy, escape from intolerable stresses, and medications that numb physical and psychic pain. Going for these "gains" doesn't make us lazy or crazy. It doesn't mean we're making ourselves sick—life takes care of that— but it may explain why we find it hard to get well. On the activity/pain cycle, illness can be "healthier," in many ways, than health.

There is a better way, though. We can change the aspects of life that damage us, and we can adapt to or escape the things we cannot change. When we are being abused at work, home, or in between, or when we abuse ourselves, our bodies tend to get sick. When we change those situations,

attitudes, or behaviors, we'll feel better, our immune and self-repair systems will work better, and usually our health will get better, although how much better varies widely. It won't happen all at once, but we can get out of the activity/sickness horror show.

They Can Wait…

This book is full of great stories meant to inspire or instruct in some way. They can wait, though. Let me start with my own experience—even if it is less spectacular than some of the other stories—because it is the source of the book. Twelve years ago, I was diagnosed with multiple sclerosis (MS) following ten years of unexplained symptoms. Before my diagnosis, I ran around like a headless chicken, and not just any chicken. I was Super Headless Chicken, committed to raising two children, splitting housework with my wife, Aisha, working as a nurse, improving my neighborhood, saving the environment, developing a songwriting career, and some more goals I can't remember now. With such divided loyalties, I naturally did a rather poor job at all of them.

In 1989, I developed extreme weakness in my right leg, then loss of vision in both eyes. At first, I tried to tough it out, because I didn't want to change my life routine. It took me five years and two more MS attacks to accept my new reality and start paying attention to my body, but finally I got with the self-care program. First, I rested; I listened to relaxation and guided-imagery tapes that helped me learn what my body needed. Its message was pretty simple: Do one thing at a time. Get help. Breathe. You can go a long way with those three instructions, and gradually I learned to get moving again, according to my body's rhythms.

I made changes, starting with exercise, a gentle form of yoga, which I now do twice a day, and gradually adding swimming and weightlifting. I cut back to part-time work and started meditating daily. (Fortunately, my family supported me through these changes.)

I got help from doctors. I never used the high-tech injectables that slow the progression in some cases of MS. They weren't approved for my type of MS, and I felt the costs, side effects, and hassle outweighed the modest benefits claimed by manufacturers. My neurologist has supported these decisions, even while prescribing those meds for other patients who

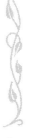

wanted them. I take one medication to control symptoms, along with supplements and an over-the-counter medicine (aspirin) that makes sense to me. At various times, I have pursued alternative treatments and used other self-care techniques, as I'll describe later.

As the years have passed, my MS so far has progressed, but very slowly, perhaps because my life is getting better. I have new symptoms, but also new abilities and strengths. I am probably in my best shape ever—admittedly, that isn't saying much—and my days are so full of love and happiness it's disgusting (at least most days). I have learned to forgive others and myself, to accept what life gives, and to be more open with people but to stand up for myself, even if I sometimes have to do it sitting down. I sincerely believe that my self-care program has contributed to the relative stability of my MS and that my response to MS has improved the quality of my life. I know how lucky I am to be able to say that.

♠ A Nursing Perspective

My twenty-five years as a nurse helped me make sense of my situation and find ways forward. In nursing, we're grounded in the scientific approach to medicine but trained to see that people's health cannot be separated from the entirety of their lives. This book largely reflects a nursing view, one that gives full importance to genetics and biochemistry but also to the practical, emotional, and spiritual dimensions of individual lives and the interactions among all of these factors.

In my work as a nurse and health coach, I spend time with hundreds of people with a variety of health conditions. I got the idea for this book when I realized that most of them, at all levels of health, weren't doing nearly as well as they could. Not only my patients but my coworkers were living with pain and unhappiness, and they often seemed too worn down, angry, careless, or hopeless to take care of themselves.

I wondered how I had come to be one of the most productive and positive people on the job, because I had distinct memories of being miserable much of my adult life. What had changed? Was I doing something right, or was I just lucky? What factors kept my associates and patients from taking better care of themselves? Searching for answers led me to the interviews, studies, and stories that make up the body of this book.

☞ Cost/Benefit Analysis

My research and experience with self-care often came back to issues of motivation. While the medical profession attributes unhealthy behavior to our not knowing what's good for us, ignorance is only a small part of the problem. The behaviors of the most knowledgeable groups, doctors and nurses, are no better than those of others with comparable incomes. In reality, the decision to engage, or not to engage, in self-care usually results from a rational, though subconscious, cost/benefit analysis. Like any change, getting well involves time, effort, and courage; we won't attempt it if the benefits are too meager or the costs too high.

Wouldn't relief of pain, avoidance of complications, better function, and longer life be sufficient motivation? It's not that simple. Our lives, and our roles in them, include pluses and minuses, pleasures and suffering, joys and grief. Too little of the good things and too much of the bad can sharply lower our estimate of the value of wellness.

Pain also has its hidden upside. Many of us may believe we somehow deserve our pain, may let physical pain distract us from emotional pain, or may find in pain (or fatigue) our only way to take a break from constant work or to accept help. Even "feeling better" brings conflict if part of us believes we deserve to suffer, if feeling bad gets us positive attention, or if the effort involved in feeling better seems too frightening.

The things that raise the costs and lower the perceived benefits of getting well are barriers to self-care. They are often the same aspects of life that contributed to our illness in the first place. We didn't cause them, usually, but with a little help, we can solve these problems and start getting better.

⟶ *Barriers to Self-Care* ⟵

First, we need reasons to live and work at getting well. Some of us live in circumstances that make life difficult and positive experiences hard to come by. If I dread getting up and going to work and dread coming home to an angry household, why should I care about getting well? If I am lonely, tense, or in pain, with little pleasure, purpose, or security, or if I am under constant stress, why should I exercise, stop smoking, or stop taking heroin for that matter? So I can live a few years longer? Why would I want to?

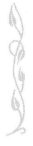

Reasons to live are plentiful, however, and most of them are cheap. People keep going for an incredible variety of motives, some of them fascinating. This is addressed in Chapter 5.

Some believe that life may be worth living, but that they, themselves, are not worth keeping alive. Low self-esteem—that is, not valuing ourselves—inhibits self-care. Many of us don't believe we can give ourselves the time and energy required to maintain our health. Everyone else's needs are more important than ours, and we don't feel we have permission to be well. We deal with getting such permission in Chapter 6.

☙ *Loss of Hope* ☙

Another demotivator is absence of hope. Why try to get well if it won't do any good? (As in, "You have less than a year to live"; "You'll never walk/run/play the xylophone again"; "Your condition is chronic and progressive. You can't get better.") Hopelessness also comes from miserable social or economic situations: "I'll never find someone to love/a place to live/a good job." It's a killer, leading to complications, suffering, and earlier death. Professionals who take away clients' sense of hope are guilty of malpractice.

Lack of self-confidence also deprives us of hope. We may disbelieve in our ability to do what we set out to do ("low self-efficacy"), or we may disbelieve that self-care will do any good. This book presents exercises for building self-efficacy, information supporting our power to help ourselves, and inspiring stories of people who have succeeded.

☙ *Resistance to Change* ☙

Fear of change raises the perceived costs of self-care. The one absolute requirement for overcoming illness is a willingness to change—if you're sick, being well is a change—but change is scary and difficult for many of us. In addition to the discomfort of changing behavior, attitude, or life situations, we may fear giving up secondary gains or fear the conflict change can bring. We may have good reasons for cherishing self-damaging habits and may want to hang onto them. Building a capacity for change is covered in Chapter 3.

⮜ *Unloving Our Bodies* ⮞

Our attitude towards our bodies affects how we see the costs and benefits of getting well. Do we enjoy and appreciate our bodies? Listen to them? Love them? If we do, we'll be much more likely to put some effort into them. If we, like most of society, regard them as machines or beasts of burden, as ugly or deficient in some way, we'll probably let them fall apart. Learning to love our bodies is taught in Chapter 7.

⮜ *Lack of Support* ⮞

Even when our motivation for wellness is high, there are a host of potential barriers. Sometimes our disease moves too fast; we can barely keep from sinking in a tide of painful change, much less think about getting well. Fortunately, such virulent conditions are rare, but if you have one, this book may not be right for you. A more common barrier is lack of support: too many demands and not enough help. Ways of slowing down and easing demands are given in Chapter 2.

Too many of us are isolated, left stranded in our highly mobile society, with few friends. Our neighbors may feel like strangers to us. Some of us are emotionally and physically distant from our families; some, many foster children, for example, never had a chance to connect with their families. Others don't know how to ask for available help, or are afraid to ask. Chapter 4 covers finding, requesting, and accepting support.

⮜ *Looking Up at the White Coats* ⮞

Getting well, like dealing with other life problems, is extremely hard for people with little education, especially for those on society's bottom rungs. Recovery requires taking some control of our lives and our care. That's a tough assignment when you have never had power over much of anything. We may have to speak up to doctors and other professionals and demand respect where little is sometimes given. This situation can be stressful enough to keep some of us from seeking help at all. Self-care requires informing ourselves, a difficult task for poor readers and for those who have been raised not to ask questions. Help in dealing with such situations is given in Chapter 6.

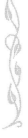

Socioeconomic factors, for many of us, cause more difficulty than the disease symptoms themselves. We have to find ways to pay for treatment, keep a roof over our heads, and care for our families. We may have to weigh time and money spent in self-care against other crucial needs, or we may simply lack convenient access to resources that could help us. We may have difficulty finding care providers familiar with our culture or language.

Some of us grew up with abusive or dysfunctional parents or care-givers who left us unloved and fearful. Others suffer from psychological problems—depression, anxiety, or worse—which make getting well appear a decidedly mixed blessing. Some of us have no role models; we've never known people who take care of themselves, so we never learned how. Such socioeconomic and psychological factors may limit, though not eliminate, self-care options.

So I don't want to hear about any of you criticizing a person with illness for not being more positive. Or about your asking someone, "Why haven't you gone back to school?" or "Why are you still depressed?" If I hear of any of you doing that, I'll come over and go upside your head with my cane. Those of us who start from harder places may have less-ambitious criteria for success. Even so, such barriers can be overcome! Given support, hope, reasons to live, and a willingness to change, there are ways forward for almost everyone.

The Riddle of Compliance

Hardly anyone decides consciously to stay sick, to keep suffering. We "for-get" to take our medicines. We are "too tired" to exercise or "too busy" to relax. We "don't get around to" writing in a journal or having that heart-to-heart discussion with our spouse about our needs. We suddenly find ourselves "craving" some food or activity we know is bad for us. We "just don't feel like" taking our blood pressure or doing our stretches today.

These acts of apparent self-sabotage tell us we've come up against a barrier to self-care. We may be thinking self-blocking thoughts (such as, "People won't like me if I take time for myself"). We may encounter practical difficulties: the roof may be leaking, the car in the shop, our mean-tempered aunt moving in with us. We may be lonely, stressed, even overwhelmed. The shame placed on people in these conflicted situations

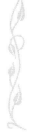

is unwarranted; such situations are part of the life difficulties that contribute to most cases of chronic illness.

We may have other, perfectly valid reasons for "noncompliance," as doctors call it when we don't follow their orders. Therapy may be too expensive, have bad side effects, be ineffective or dangerous, be too disruptive of our lives, or conflict with our values. We may also have negative reasons: rebellion against authority or unwillingness to accept that we have a problem. When faced with noncompliant patients, care providers should consider these possibilities. This book explores solutions to them.

Health-care workers who try to force healthy behaviors on us by using fear often do more harm than good. Catherine Feste, author of *The Physician Within*, developed diabetes forty years ago, at age ten, when that diagnosis usually meant a short and miserable life. She says, "I can't imagine taking the prevention approach. I can't see myself getting out of bed in the morning, stretching, and saying, 'Well, another day to prevent blindness and kidney failure!' As if that were a reason to live!" Feste has thrived with her diabetes, she believes, because she has found meaningful and enjoyable things to do with her life, not because of fear of the consequences of failure. Each of us has the ability to follow her inspiring model. We just need to learn ways over the barriers.

Why We Need Doctors

Self-care doesn't mean rejecting medicine. Working effectively with health professionals (Chapters 4, 6, and 10) can make all the difference in getting well. This book is no substitute for medical care or for educating ourselves about our particular condition. I'm not saying this to avoid getting sued; medical treatment helps in most conditions, and it's getting more helpful all the time. Good doctors or nurses will share with us what they know. Medical tests can help us understand what is happening and monitor our progress. We nearly always need doctors—and often other healers—on our health-care team.

However, I know of no chronic condition where medical care can effect a cure all by itself, or where the doctor's contribution is more important than the patient's. Too often, expensive and invasive treatments of dubious value distract a patient from self-care measures that could be

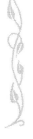

much more helpful. Coronary artery bypass surgery frequently falls into this category, if it takes the place of relaxation, exercise, healthy eating, and social support (the program developed by Dean Ornish). So does indiscriminate use of antidepressants, if they take the place of exercise, positive self-talk, and counseling. In some conditions where causes and treatment are poorly understood, such as fibromyalgia, irritable bowel syndrome, chronic fatigue, and certain autoimmune conditions, the search for currently nonexistent medical answers can delay self-care measures more likely to improve our situation.

Overcoming illness means cooperating with doctors, not attacking them. Most are overworked and underappreciated and will welcome sharing responsibility with their patients. (If they don't, we can find others who will.) "Self-management" programs have been shown to reduce doctor visits, hospitalizations, and medication use, saving resources better used elsewhere. We don't do our doctors any favors by giving them too much power. They cannot heal us without our participation. Self-care is a winning proposition for everyone involved.

☞ Recovery, Yes; Cure, Maybe

This book applies a recovery model to getting well. Like a twelve-step program, it promises a lifelong strategy for living well, not a cure. I still have MS; Cindy Wong still has hypertension and thyroid problems; Rob Mitchell, quoted at the beginning of this chapter, still has AIDS. I can guarantee that if you read twenty self-help books and follow all the advice contained in this book and given by your doctor, you will still die, eventually.

What counts, though, is what we do with the time we have, and the knowledge in this book can empower anyone to live a richer, healthier life, to take better care of themselves, and to work better with others. These skills sometimes lead to cure—more often, however, they do not—but whatever our condition, we can always feel better, more well, more fully alive. We may also wind up as more fulfilled people who tend to bring happiness and inspiration to those we meet or at least to annoy them by being so cheerful.

Doctors have long known that an arthritic person's level of pain and disability has almost no correlation with the amount of joint damage visible on X ray. Neurologists have found that MS patients' symptoms bear only a slight relation to the scars seen in their brains on an MRI. The whole person is much more than the disease.

Doctors and educators at Stanford University have developed a program, the Chronic Disease Self-Management Program, which Kaiser Permanente now presents as Healthier Living (HL). This program, which I sometimes facilitate, aims to help people manage their own conditions and lives. The results, proven repeatedly, include higher self-rated health, less disability, less limitation in social and role activities, increased energy, fewer doctor visits and hospitalizations, and less distress. Yet, participants' conditions have usually not changed much clinically.

☞ How to Use This Book

Each chapter of this book presents knowledge to help with specific areas of self-care. No one needs all of it, so feel free to jump around to what seems most relevant to you. You may even want to go straight to Chapter 9, which presents steps for developing a personal self-care plan.

Self-help exercises and resources for material covered in each chapter have been placed in their own sections at the back of the book. You may want to read the book through once and then go back to the parts that seem right for you and try the related exercises.

The Art of Getting Well reflects the work and lives of hundreds of people who try to live fully and to make this world a better place. I hope you find within these pages the help, information, inspiration, or at least the entertainment value you are looking for.

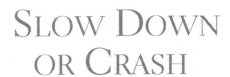

SLOW DOWN
OR CRASH

Rest is the basis of all healing.

Father Thomas Keating

AT THE SPEED MOST OF US LIVE, we don't have time to figure out where we are headed. Cajun psychologist Wayne Sotile tells this story to illustrate "the difference between going 30 and 130":

Mrs. Boudreau hears an emergency announcement on the radio. There's a crazy man driving the wrong way on the freeway. She immediately calls her husband's car phone.

"Boudreau," she says, "if you're on the freeway, you got to get off. The radio says there's a crazy man driving the wrong way."

"Call 'em back," yells Boudreau. "Tell 'em there ain't just one. There's hundreds of 'em!"

This chapter explores a crucial step in getting well: getting out of the Boudreau lane, slowing down, saving some energy for healing, and increasing awareness of our bodies, surroundings, and feelings. Awareness results when we give more attention to what we see, hear, smell, touch, and feel, and less to the endless tape of worries and babble put out by society and our own verbal brains.

In an economy and culture driven by hurry, too many of us are running at Boudreau's unsafe speed. The constant tension, the endless tasks to complete, the SOS messages we hear all day can fill life with too much pain and anxiety to make wellness worthwhile. In fact, they provide powerful reasons to get sick.

Sickness has the ability to make us rest, whether our conscious minds want to or not. Lying still after an operation or a heart attack, cut off from our usual pressures and demands, gives us an opportunity to take a long, slow look at our lives. A slower pace brought on by a disabling condition like MS or arthritis can allow us to smell the flowers, feel the sunshine, and relax our bodies into healthier states.

I wouldn't count on it, though, because slowing down even because of illness or disability is by no means automatic. At one holistic-health conference, I saw a woman dashing madly down a path, apparently worried about being late for the next workshop on relaxation. The striking thing was that she was blind, clearly risking a collision or a fall, her cane whistling wildly about.

Folk wisdom says that illness is Nature's way of getting us to slow down. Maybe Nature needs another way, because this one isn't working. You might think a diagnosis of hypertension would get us to relax. More often, though, even the first chest pain won't do it; it takes a stroke or a couple of heart attacks. Hurry is built so deeply into our culture and consciousness that it takes an explosion to uproot it.

☞ "I Don't Have Time, I Don't Have Time"

Typical is Beth's story. This intelligent, educated, attractive woman tried to fight her illness for years, spending all her time and money pursuing a cure before realizing that no treatment would work until she stopped rushing and learned to relax. Beth was a recovering alcoholic in her mid-thirties with a fledgling family-therapy practice when she gradually started losing energy. Eventually, getting out of bed became a difficult chore.

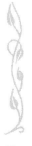

After some months, she was diagnosed with chronic fatigue syndrome (CFS). Many experts now believe CFS is caused by a combination of an immune-system malfunction, viral infection—three different pathogenic viruses were found in Beth's blood—and psychological factors. As such, it is a perfect example of how harmful aspects of the environment, combined with our conscious and unconscious responses, can make us sick.

Just getting her career going, Beth wasn't thinking about slowing down. "I just kept on working, thinking that it would pass. I would see my clients, and I would take breaks after I'd seen maybe a couple, and I would totally collapse," she remembers. After her diagnosis came the frantic search for effective treatment.

"About a year later," she remembers, "we were trying different medications—gamma globulin injections, all the other things they were doing then—and at one point they said antidepressants had worked well. I tried a couple of different antidepressants and nothing happened. Then at the end of 1989 I was prescribed Prozac, and just like that, miraculously, the entire thing disappeared. Totally disappeared, every single symptom."

Don't assume that because an antidepressant drug relieved Beth's symptoms, her illness was "all in her head." Quite the opposite, it demonstrates how tightly mind and body are connected. This class of medicines, the selective serotonin reuptake inhibitors (SSRIs), has proven helpful in many physical conditions. In most illnesses, though, relief by drugs is only temporary, if damaging ways of life go unchanged.

After finding the Prozac cure, Beth felt free to go back to the behaviors that were contributing to her illness. "For a year and a half I was symptom free, and that's when I really dug in and started building my practice. In that period of time I built a huge practice and was working from early morning till late night. In late 1991, I started to notice some of the symptoms coming back. By the end of '91, all the symptoms were back, but one thing that I was unable to do, which everybody was recommending, was slow down. I used up every ounce of energy I had, because I didn't want to lose what I'd built. I kept telling myself, 'I don't have time, I don't have time, I don't have time.'"

~ *Mantra of Death* ~

I call the phrase "I don't have time," which all of us repeat at some point, the mantra of death. We tell ourselves we are running out of time, which really only happens when we die. We can take a great weight off our minds and bodies by saying, when we feel rushed, "I have plenty of time for every-thing." If that sounds too unrealistic, try, "I have time for the things that matter." Repeat as often as necessary, because actually we do have time for the important things. It's the trivial stuff that makes us crazy. At this point in my life I never say, "I don't have time" for this or that, not even once. I say, "I have other things to do" or "I need to rest" or simply "I don't want to" or "no."

~ Time's Bullet Train

Our society tends to view time as a speeding train that we either catch or that leaves us behind (or runs us over). Every day, we have to chase it down and catch it again. It's worth noting that most cultures and peoples throughout history have not shared this view of time. Farming people see time as a circle, going round and round, coming back to the same places each day and each year—a view in which minutes and seconds aren't so crucial. Even more peacefully, pre-agricultural people tended to see time as a lake. We simply move around in time—through the mornings and afternoons and evenings—but we have all we want; it isn't going any-where. Obviously, if we live in the lake of time all the time, we will miss a lot of appointments. But if we live on the bullet train of time all the time, we will reach our final destination, death, far too fast, and we won't see much of the scenery.

Beth wasn't ready to get off the train, illness or no. Refusing to make room for rest, she went back to searching for a cure, this time in the alternative-health world. She got walked on by massage practitioners and took all kinds of supplements and cleansing treatments. It wasn't until she had spent all her money and gone into debt that she remembered the serenity prayer ("Grant me the serenity to accept the things I cannot change, the courage to change the things I can, and the wisdom to know the difference") from her days in AA.

Beth decided to forget what seemed beyond her power and to go about changing what she could: the pace and complexity of her life. She says the message of her illness was one word: "Simplify!" When she started simplifying and slowing down by following some of the methods described later in this chapter, her life gradually became more manageable and successful. Her symptoms have not disappeared, but they are under control, and she enjoys her career, her family, and a full and rewarding life. She rides her bike along the shore for exercise, pleasure, and transportation.

You might expect an illness named "chronic fatigue" to respond well to rest, but most other conditions do, too. Relaxation methods of various types have proven effective in improving function and reducing symptoms in virtually every chronic condition studied.

Get Ahead of the Curve

Unless we are physically and mentally sedentary, complete couch potatoes (or in some cases severely depressed), we can probably benefit from slowing down. It's a question of energy. We each have a supply of energy, a level that can be increased with various health practices but will always be limited. That energy has to serve us for work, social and mental activities, growth, and also for our bodies' healing and maintenance. I believe that if we give all our energy to work, worry, and other demands, our bodies' defense and repair systems won't have enough energy to do their job. If we want to get well, we have to save some life force for our bodies.

Many people refuse to cut back at all. Others will reduce their schedules to accommodate health problems, but only by the minimum amount possible. In fact, to effect real change it may be possible to keep working, say, thirty-five hours a week, but only if we give up everything else. If we do not cut back somewhere, our health will continue to deteriorate, we will grudgingly cut back more, and pretty soon we're totally disabled. That's the curve of chronic illness without self-care.

We need to get ahead of the curve. What does this mean? Cut back work to twenty hours if at all possible. Consider taking disability, at least temporarily; let some other things go; do whatever must be done to get time and energy for healing. I'm not talking about time just to lie around vegetating—activity is important, too—but rather time to find

help, connect with our bodies, figure out how to make our lives work. When we get sick, either we can take the opportunity to stop and listen to our bodies (see Chapter 7) or we can try to muscle through, charging along the path that childhood programming and social demands have set for us. If we choose the latter option, we shouldn't be surprised when our bodies come back and hit us again, harder.

Living on the Dog Track

We don't usually need to stop everything we're doing, but we do need to relax. For many of us life feels like a dog track, where we live like greyhounds chasing mechanical rabbits (such as money, happiness, or doing good), while simultaneously being stuck from behind with cattle prods (such as fear of poverty or low self-esteem). The race runs through our waking hours and often invades our sleep. We fear that the ever rising tide of responsibilities will overwhelm us if we slack off even momentarily or that we will miss some vital opportunity for advancement or growth. Meanwhile, the pain builds in our organs and muscles, the healing systems start to wear down, and next thing we know the doctor is recommending a triple bypass.

Let's put all the rabbits and cattle prods together and label them stress. The word *stress* has several meanings, but in common usage it means anything that results in what psychologist Walter Cannon called the fight or flight response. The stress response actually involves release of more than thirty hormones, neurotransmitters, and other chemicals that temporarily make us more alert, energetic, stronger, and faster. This chemical mix, which includes endorphins (our natural painkillers), makes stress feel good in controlled doses, explaining the popularity of roller coasters, deadlines, and other stressful activities.

The stress response gives us tense muscles and rapid breathing and heartbeat, while suppressing other bodily functions not used for fight or flight, including our digestive and immune systems. It's really a wonderful survival tool in small doses—when facing a ravenous wild animal, say—but today many of us stay stressed all day long at the thought of arriving two minutes late for an appointment or at the memory of a slightly strained conversation with a spouse.

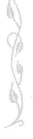

✐ What's Wrong with Stress?

Research confirms that excess stress worsens nearly every health condition. Stress raises cholesterol levels and blood pressure, and it makes blood clot faster, causing heart attacks and strokes. It cripples immune function, making us more susceptible to infections and tumors. It raises blood sugar levels in diabetics, makes irritable bladders more difficult to control and increases inflammation. It triggers lupus attacks, causes premature births, and increases pain and disability in arthritis. Nearly identical reactions occur in animals experimentally subjected to stress, so it's not all in our heads. Prolonged stress is a killer, and rushed, unaware living is a major cause of stress.

More to the point, too much stress makes us feel miserable. Our muscles get tight, our breathing short. We develop pains in various parts of our body, and we feel tired all the time. This kind of stress takes the pleasure out of life and leaves us on the constant edge of anger or depression. When we feel this way we are much less likely to engage in self-care.

It must be said that some people can suffer very little stress and still be sick. Some of us are actually understressed, bored, doing little or nothing to keep ourselves interested in life. This is a less common situation; ways out of it involve getting ourselves moving through exercise or reengaging life through some of the suggestions in Chapter 5.

✐ Stop and Take a Breath

How do we slow down when we are surrounded by a rat race? How do we relax our muscles and our internal organs—give our bodies space and time to heal—when we have the demands of others and our own worries jacking us up? How do we gain awareness? Watching news on TV or lying in bed, body tense, mind racing through everything we've done wrong that week, won't do it. We can be lying still and not relaxing.

Instead, we start by taking a couple of deep breaths.

Since we don't think about breathing, we often don't notice when, under stress, we are exchanging the absolute minimum amount of air. When we don't breathe deeply enough, we tend to tense up. We can't think straight or relax, and then our breathing gets worse in a vicious cycle.

We can easily break the cycle by stopping for a few deep, slow breaths, breathing into our tense backs and abdomens, and paying attention to the way our breath moves. I emphasize doing one thing at a time because whatever else we are doing we also have to breathe at the same time.

Breathing exercises are discussed in Chapter 9, but more important is paying attention to breathing throughout the day so we don't get so stressed in the first place. Certain activities, such as talking, lend themselves to forgetting to breathe properly. Eating can also interfere with breathing, especially for those of us who rush from one bite to the next. Taking breath breaks between bites will help your digestion, your energy level, and your appreciation of food.

We all tend to hold our breath when we're afraid. If we pay attention we might note other times when we aren't breathing enough—for example, while driving in traffic, brushing our teeth, trying to meet a deadline at work, or being nice to someone we would desperately like to punch out. In all cases, taking a few deep breaths, with awareness, will calm our body and mind. I try to use all of these situations as cues to breathe, and I encourage you to do the same. When you get angry or frustrated, breathe. When the light turns red or after you take the first bite of a meal, take a deep breath or two. As of this writing air is still free, so use as much as you want!

⸺ *Conscious Breathing* ⸺

Conscious breathing, that is, paying deliberate attention to the process of breathing, is the beginning of what is usually called meditation. If the idea of meditation still seems weird, foreign, difficult, or frightening, then call it "the relaxation response," as Dr. Herbert Benson did in his groundbreaking 1975 book of the same name. Or you can call it "just sitting there," or "just being," as some personal coaches say. You don't have to call it anything, really; just do it!

Breathing becomes meditation when we start to pay attention to the actual process: the air moving through the nose and throat, the abdomen expanding, muscles relaxing, or any other part. The idea is to allow the mind to become quiet by giving it something to center on: the breath, a single word like "one," or an object or concept.

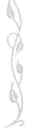

Father Thomas Keating teaches a similar practice called "centering prayer," which involves focusing on one object or word. Prayer, when done in this peaceful way, yields benefits fully equivalent to those of meditation or other relaxation practices. Many people combine them. A woman with severe arthritis told me, "Prayer is talking to God; meditation is listening to him"—a formula that clearly indicates how the two can go together.

⟡ Other Slowing-Down Techniques

Dozens of other relaxation techniques also work. Peaceful music or recorded nature sounds are widely used and highly effective, as are techniques centering around the progressive relaxation of muscles. All kinds of relaxation tapes are sold at bookstores and health-food stores, and they're not all New Age California hippie stuff. Or you can keep it simple: Have a picnic. Go watch the birds. Take a nap once in a while. Actually, anything that puts us more in touch with nature or with our bodies, even if we are in pain, tends to be relaxing.

Diane Ulmer, R.N., who worked with Dr. Myron Friedman, author of *Type-A Behavior and Your Heart,* has more ideas. Among them: Drive in the slow lane (or take the bus!). Practice listening to others without interrupting. Take your watch off. Stand in the slow line and use your mind creatively to take advantage of the wait. That last one sounds crazy when you first hear it, but since we have so much enforced waiting in our society, we can choose to make it a frustration or a chance to relax. Use the time for some deep breathing, exercise, or meeting people. Nurse Ulmer likes to say, "We are human beings, not human doings." We don't have to be producing or accomplishing every waking minute to justify our existence.

Physical activity can also be relaxing. It's usually better to go for a walk than to lie in bed stewing over our problems. Yoga and tai chi (see Chapter 9) are both relaxing and energizing. If we pay attention to our surroundings, our bodies, and our breathing, mild exercise can relax us quite well.

⟜ *Remember the Sabbath* ⟝

God thought it was so important for us to rest one day a week that he put it into the Ten Commandments. In fact, working on the Sabbath was among the dozens of offenses punishable by death in Old Testament law, which tells us how important the Israelites thought it was and also how much coercion was required to get people to comply. Unfortunately, few of us, even those who attend religious services on the Sabbath, actually take that day to rest. Don't worry, though. Consistently working seven days a week without a break will, in fact, tend to make you die sooner, so maybe it all works out.

Religious counselor and author Wayne Muller says the Sabbath is a day to "delight in creation, and to give thanks for the blessings we may have missed in our preoccupation with our work. It is a time to remember and celebrate what is beautiful and sacred." Taking a weekly Sabbath day to rest and renew is like leaving a field fallow to renew its productivity. It sets us up for the week ahead.

Overstressing is a habit, and so is relaxing. They cannot coexist. If we practice relaxation or meditation on a regular basis during the week and take a weekly Sabbath day, our bodies will feel better. Pain and fatigue, and sometimes other symptoms as well, will decrease; energy levels and pleasure will increase. Often, disease processes will slow—though this is not guaranteed—because our bodies will be getting the oxygen and rest they need to heal.

Why aren't stress-reduction techniques more widely used in medicine? Good research shows that relaxation programs are as effective and cheaper than most cardiac drugs and have the added side effect of making us feel better. In a large study of people who'd suffered heart attacks, 30 percent of those given regular medical treatment had another attack, bypass surgery, or stroke within five years, 20 percent of those on medical treatment plus exercise had another event, but only 9 percent of those whose care included a stress-reduction program did so! That is a two-thirds reduction in life-threatening events, yet such programs are still barely mentioned in most medical books or treatment guidelines. Perhaps relaxation programs need the marketing department of a large pharmaceutical company in order to get doctors to prescribe them.

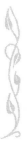

~ *Awareness Is Its Own Reward* ~

Living with awareness, a practice that in essence is a side effect of slowing down and relaxing, offers benefits that extend beyond our physical health. By paying attention to our surroundings and our state of mind and body, we can tune in to our environment and learn what helps us and what hurts. We can appreciate, enjoy, and get to know the plants and animals, the sun and rain. We can pay more attention to other people. People who learn these skills find that other folks really like being around them, a nice switch for some of us.

One of Dr. Herbert Benson's patients reported, "Not only has [relaxation] made me more relaxed physically and mentally, but...I seem to have become calmer, more open and receptive...more patient, overcoming some fears. I am stronger physically and mentally. I take better care of myself.... I really enjoy it, too!"

Awareness of our own bodies helps to prevent pain and to increase comfort. How often do we ignore a minor backache or headache until it turns into a huge one? How often do we keep eating a certain food, ignoring little stomach cramps and twinges only to feel awful later?

Living without awareness is like buying a ticket to a movie and then not watching it. After all, we live on a planet that not only feeds and shelters us, but puts on light shows in the sky and art exhibits in the gardens and landscapes. But somehow, we often manage to avoid seeing them. Awareness also has the wonderful capacity to slow down time. When it feels like your life is rushing by you, perhaps you are rushing by it instead. If we don't see the flowers, taste the food, or get to know the people around us, it's not really their fault, is it? No wonder time seems to speed up as we age; we throw away many of our minutes, hours, and days.

Charles Kuralt, who chronicled the byways of the United States in his TV show *On the Road*, said, "Thanks to the interstate highway system, it is now possible to travel across the country from coast to coast, without seeing anything." Sadly, many of us live exactly that way, racing from birth coast to death coast without experiencing much of the trip. Unawareness wastes our lives as well as our health.

To see how elastic time can be, how much time you really have, try counting each breath as you inhale and exhale, slowly and with awareness. (This is sort of a beginner's meditation.) Other thoughts will come to you,

but just let them go without giving them your attention. Keep bringing your attention back to the breathing and counting. By the time you get to ten, you'll feel like you've been sitting there for twenty minutes, and you'll feel good. Try paying full attention to your lover's touch or to the taste of an apple—or to anything else—just a couple times a day. I guarantee your life will slow way down. You'll also be more relaxed, less stressed, and, therefore in all probability, healthier.

Brother, Can You Spare Ten Minutes?

Sometimes our financial and housing situations are precarious, noisy, and uncomfortable. Though a mere ten minutes of relaxation twice a day produces tremendous benefit, even that little time can be difficult to come by. It's hard to meditate when the kids are screaming and the boom boxes are thumping, the neighbors arguing, the bills mounting, and the pots and pans rattling. How do we find the time to rest and gain awareness in all that mess?

Remember that there are twenty-four hours in a day. There are doors to close, earplugs to wear. Don't answer your phone (at least not during meals or rest periods)—that's what answering machines are for. Turn the ringer off; you can listen to the message later. Stop watching the TV news; do we really need to know who killed whom today? Chances are, if we put our minds to it, we can find ten minutes twice a day to relax.

If the household is noisy, try giving ten minutes notice. "Listen up, everyone! In ten minutes, I'm closing the door and doing my relaxation. Don't disturb me unless it's a real emergency." Use the ten-minute pre-relaxation period to put out any household brushfires that might flare while you're relaxing, and write down a list of things you need to do later so worrying about them doesn't interfere.

We may have lots of housework, child care, and other responsibilities, but many household tasks can be turned into relaxation opportunities. Relatively mindless jobs such as washing dishes or mopping can actually increase our energy if we treat them as a meditation. Really focus on them—or on breathing—instead of worrying about getting them done faster. One of my Healthier Living participants with arthritis tried this method. "It takes a little longer," she told me, "but I have more energy, and things are just as clean."

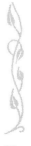

29

If conditions around the home are too crazy, learn to speak up. Above all else, get help! Having someone watch the kids, do housework, take you to a park, or keep the household quiet for half an hour once a day can make all the difference. (Getting help from others and becoming assertive enough to get our own needs met are covered in more detail in later chapters, particularly Chapter 4.)

⚓ *What Really Counts?* ⚓

What do you do with the familiar feeling that there's "so much to do and so little time"? First of all, remind yourself that the bigger the task or the longer the journey the slower you have to go. Important things take time. In a hundred-yard dash, you run as hard as you can to the finish line, then you collapse. Life isn't like that; it's a marathon. You have to pace yourself. We can learn to organize our time better, but more important is learning to focus on what's really important, as Beth did.

When we left Beth, she was dragging through the day with chronic fatigue syndrome dogging her steps, but still trying to do it all. Things started going better for her when she began working to simplify her life.

As Beth told me, "My methods for slowing down and simplifying extend to every area of my life. I've simplified my wardrobe. What's important to me now is that I feel I look good without wearing too many pieces or trying to impress people. Food is another area where I've simplified. I don't worry about making fancy meals; I just enjoy simple nutritious food based on a healthy food plan I can live with. I periodically go through every possession and ask myself, 'Does this cost me more energy than I get from it?' If it does, I change it or get rid of it."

Everyone needs to set priorities, but health problems can really up the ante. A lot of things we treat as necessities are actually optional, and we can conserve energy for ourselves by letting them go. Is *Better Homes and Gardens* coming over for a photo shoot today? If not, maybe cleaning behind the refrigerator can wait. Do we really have to go to the next town to buy from a particular hardware store or bakery? Do we need to go to that meeting we know will be a waste of time? Do we really need another car or a bigger home?

⟿ *The Magic Word: "No"* ⟿

And do we really need to be doing for others with every bit of energy we have? I've lost count of the number of people who have told me how they wore down their own health caring for relatives or keeping things together for the whole family, only to find out that nobody appreciated their sacrifice. One woman with diabetes said, "Right before I was diagnosed with hypertension, my nineteen-year-old daughter and I had a big blow up. She was blaming me for everything that had happened in the past. I kind of sat back and said to myself, 'I gave my life for her, and she's not appreciating me, so something is wrong with this picture.'"

Other people, especially children, have valid demands on our time, but it is vital that we reserve some time and energy for ourselves. When we're kids, the magic words are "please" and "thank you." When we get older, the magic word is "no." In every Healthier Living (HL) class, students consistently bring up the importance of saying "no" and sticking to it. One HL participant, Danielle, told me, "I never used to say no, but people are really okay with it after the initial shock. My son actually congratulated me for protecting myself."

I'm not suggesting that we become totally selfish and ignore others' needs, but simply that we include our own needs somewhere near the top of the list. The question of when, how, and why to say no keeps coming up in this book because everyone with a chronic condition has to deal with it (see Chapters 4 and 6).

We also must learn to refuse some well-intended offers. Friends and family may not readily accept our need for rest, particularly if we have a condition that doesn't show on the outside. "But you look fine! Let's go shopping," someone may say. We may have to answer, "No, thanks for asking, though. Maybe we can do it another time, soon."

⟿ The Day Superman Rested

It's not always other people's needs and wants that make us crazy. Just as often, our own desires—for material possessions, recognition, power, or personal growth—cause us to overwork and drive our bodies like beasts of

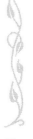

burden. We don't just burn our candles at both ends; we vaporize them with a blowtorch! Sometimes we find ourselves wanting to have, do, and be more when what we really need is to rest. The kind of selfishness this book recommends involves taking care of ourselves, not going after things that cost far more money, time, and energy than they are worth.

Even among activities that seem valuable, we may find it necessary to focus. We can only do so many things in our lives, certainly at any one time. If we limit our commitments, we usually find we do a much better job with the ones we keep—and we also have more energy and time for self-care.

We have good social and psychological reasons for living as if we were possessed of superpowers. We tend to define our self-worth by our accomplishments, feeling that if we are not doing something productive, we are worthless. Some of us hold a belief that nothing good can happen without us. Others keep up a frantic pace to ward off depression. In the latter case, therapy, exercise, or medication may help. All of us need to recognize and change the harmful ideas driving our hyperactivity, even if we require professional help to do it. We have to turn in the Superman costumes before we hit the kryptonite wall.

Though slowing down is often an indispensable starting point in getting well, it's rarely the whole answer. We usually also must change one or more aspects of our lives. Change often seems scary and difficult; learning how and why to make changes is the topic of the next chapter.

MAKE A CHANGE,
ANY CHANGE

What is the message pain tries to convey? Most commonly,
it has to do with the process of change.

Dr. David Bresler

HEALTH PROBLEMS AND SYMPTOMS, with the possible exception of purely genetic disorders, carry a signal to change our lives. Even the flu tells us to rest and take vitamin C. The message can be as obvious as "Get better shoes," if our feet hurt, or it may be harder to decipher. It might relate to an internal issue—such as our fatigue telling us, "Stop trying to be the perfect mother, already!" Or it could be alerting us to the need for an external change—such as our asthma telling us, "Get the mold out of this apartment, or move away!" Changing harmful situations such as these makes it possible to get well.

I learned a great lesson last year about the power of life change. My teacher was a bit unusual in that it was green and nearly silent. In fact, it was a rubber plant, one that had had a bad childhood. The plant's previous owner had kept it in a dim corner for years, so it had grown twisted, trying to get sunlight. Its trunk gradually became so bent that the slightest touch could send the plant toppling over, spilling dirt on the floor.

The strain of fighting gravity eventually wore the plant down, as hard lives will do, and it became infected with no fewer than three fungi or molds. It had white spots, gray patches, and black growths on every leaf. When I took some leaves to the nursery for diagnosis, the staff said, "Don't bring those things in here! They'll infect our whole stock!" They sold me some antifungal spray, but advised me to throw out this plant to protect the others.

I did put it out for one day, but something made me reconsider. Along with MS, I have severe scoliosis, a marked twist of the spine that bends me to the left. Perhaps I identified with that twisted, long-ignored plant. So I brought it in and stripped off all the leaves except one, the least infected. Without much hope, I washed the whole thing down with the antifungal liquid. I moved the plant to my bedroom and, so it wouldn't fall over, placed it so that the bend in the trunk leaned against the edge of my writing desk.

For the first time in its life, the plant was supported. And it took off. Within three weeks that thing had so many big, beautiful, healthy leaves it didn't look like the same plant. Even the diseased leaf got better, although it's not quite as pretty as the ones that had never been sick. It's still growing furiously, as if to make up for lost time; and it's still twisted, but now it's perhaps the healthiest plant in the apartment.

Of course, that rubber tree is just a plant. But how many people have grown up in dark corners, twisting themselves into weird shapes trying to find some love? How many become sick or suffer simply because they lack support? And how many, even with a major illness, could grow spectacularly if they made a few life changes?

☞ Change = Life

AIDS activists have a slogan: "Silence = death." They not only mean that people with AIDS must fight for more services, better care, and more research, but also that they cannot let their disease make them passive or hopeless. In my nursing practice I have seen many people with hepatitis or AIDS whose fights to make changes in the system have inspired them to change their own lives. These people frequently go into remission and live positively for decades.

When people have an incurable illness, pain, poverty, or some other form of loss and suffering, they are frequently told to accept it. We do need to accept, but we also need to change damaging conditions that are within our power to change. My friend Julie, a devout Christian, lived with two chronic problems: disabling neck pain and her nasty ex-husband, Jim, who derided her to her children, threatened her, and interfered with her finances every chance he got. She never fought back. Her attitude towards Jim was tolerance; she regarded his harassment as a test and believed "God would take care of it." I suggested that if God loved her he did not want to give this jerk a free pass to torment her. After her pastor gave her the same message, she got a lawyer to put some limits on her ex's behavior, and her neck pain improved enough that she could return to work.

☞Any Change At All

We usually think of health changes in terms of diet, exercise, rest, and the like, but the whole range of life factors comes into play in getting well. These modifications can be huge decisions, like leaving a miserable relationship, or simple choices, like getting a better mattress to sleep on or cutting down on coffee. Even small changes can produce large payoffs. By giving us a sense of control, they set the stage for further growth. It doesn't always matter much what change we decide to make. Just doing something—anything—for ourselves or for our bodies makes a huge difference. In this chapter, we'll start with changing ourselves—behaviors, habits, and attitudes—and then cover changing harmful conditions in our lives, especially in the areas of work, relationships, and housing.

Several recent studies have confirmed the power of "self-efficacy," the feeling that we can do what we set out to do. Self-efficacy has been positively linked with lower rates of hospitalization, higher self-reported health, and greater longevity and quality of life. Most of us don't really believe in our efficacy, though, until we actually change something about our lives and see some results. The sooner we make a change, the sooner we feel effective, and the better off we are.

And here's the really good news: It doesn't matter where you start. Say you were out of shape and depressed. You could probably think of five or six changes that might help move your life to a better track, and they

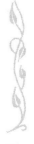

would all work (except dieting; that rarely works). It wouldn't matter if you started psychotherapy, exercise, meditation, healthier eating, bird watching, attending college, or playing the flügelhorn. I would choose exercise, but you might pick something else, maybe something not on my list.

Asthma is a good example of a condition for which different changes work for different people. Asthma, more than most diseases, responds to environmental change. A gas heater, dirty rugs, mold, or air pollution, among other factors, can make an asthmatic's life miserable, so cleaning up or getting away from such problems can greatly improve health. Other people with asthma respond better to stress reduction, relaxation, and breathing exercises—usually along with medication—because asthma is largely a stress response to environmental irritants. A doctor I know who has mild asthma developed a terrible asthmatic reaction to cats after a painful divorce from his cat-loving wife. A couple of times after visiting a room in which a cat had recently been, he needed adrenaline to stop his wheezing. (He didn't need to see the cat or even to know of its existence to have the reaction. His body knew.) Through the use of psychotherapy, he got a better handle on his grief over the divorce, and the asthmatic reactions stopped. Now he can pet or play with a cat without difficulty.

⌒ How Change Works

To help us survive as a species when life was much more dangerous than it is now, our brains learned to feel comfortable with the status quo, even if it was awful. So it's normal to fear change to some degree. However, the actual process of change is pretty straightforward. Behavior-change experts say we need only three things to make change: motivation, a method, and practice. Motivation, the hard part, is covered in Chapters 5 and 6. The rest of this chapter is about method and practice. The following are the first four guidelines to affecting change:

1. The best changes are things you *want* to do, not things someone else tells you to do. In Healthier Living classes (based on the Stanford Chronic Disease Self-Management Program, or CDSMP), each member is asked to make a weekly action plan. One woman, Martha,

planned for three weeks in a row to do more walking, but she never did it. Finally the truth came out. She told us, "I don't really like to walk; I just thought I should." Substituting another form of exercise got her going.

2. You need to believe that whatever change you plan to make will actually help. If you need convincing, you can talk with others who share your issues, read books and articles, and/or listen to your doctor to obtain evidence of your idea's effectiveness.

3. Changes should be realistically attainable. People tend to want things to go too far, too fast. They turn self-care into a form of self-abuse. "I will run on the treadmill an hour a day." "I want to lose a hundred pounds in six months, like that person on the TV ad." Good luck! We have much better chances if we make changes that feel good as we go along, and if we set realistic timetables.

4. Start small, breaking large goals into achievable chunks. If your goal is finding a better job, list the many smaller changes you might need to make and the resources you will need to accomplish them—and plan to take them on one at a time. It is far better to start with a less ambitious goal and achieve it than to shoot for some gigantic transformation and fall short. The first pattern leaves you feeling good about yourself and ready for more; the second makes you want to forget the whole thing.

It is amazing how rapidly we can improve if we go slowly. On the suggestion of a young trainer at the YMCA, I began using a stair-climbing machine at a time when I could barely climb one flight. I started with three minutes three times a week—a modest goal. I increased the time by an average of one minute (sometimes more, sometimes less) each month, which is pretty damn slow. But do the math! One year later, I was at fifteen minutes, supposedly equivalent to thirty-nine flights of stairs. I'm glad I didn't have to climb that many in real life, but I found I could also walk a lot farther on level ground. Slow (not necessarily steady) improvement will get you where you want to go.

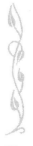

✑ *Action Planning* ✑

As its main tool, Stanford's CDSMP features the action plan: a commitment or contract with ourselves to take a specific short-term step toward larger goals. Again, the step needs to be something you want to do and reasonably can do, and it needs to be highly specific. Most people's plans for change fail through vagueness. Consider the plan, "I will exercise more." It's highly unlikely this plan will be carried out. What, specifically, are you going to do? How often? For how long? When? It's too easy to weasel out of a plan like that.

A more promising action plan would be, "I will walk for thirty minutes a day, four days this week, after dinner." You could get more specific, naming the days, with whom you will walk—if there is such a person or animal—and what you will do if it rains. The more specific the better!

In HL, we also ask people for a confidence level, on a scale of zero to ten, that they will carry out their entire plan. If they don't have a confidence level of seven or higher, we ask them to identify barriers and obstacles they think will get in the way. Then the class brainstorms possible solutions to these problems, and the person picks one that gets them to seven. Sometimes the solution is to make the goal less difficult, e.g., "I will run/walk three days a week," instead of "six days a week." Sometimes it involves getting help, e.g., "My neighbor will watch my kids for thirty minutes while I do relaxation, and I will walk her dog in exchange."

✑ *Stay Flexible* ✑

We have to be flexible about our plans. If we say we'll walk five days a week and we're snowed in by a blizzard, we have to find different ways to accomplish the goal. Perhaps we can walk in the house, do another form of exercise, or, sometimes, accept that we couldn't fulfill the plan this week, but we will next week.

The simple format for an action plan, then, is "I will do X activity, Y times this week, for Z minutes, at such and such a time, in such and such a way," not "I will try." As Yoda, the high-tech sock puppet, said in *Star Wars*, there is no "try" when it comes to behavior change. These are things that are within our power to do, and if they are not, we need to pick

something less ambitious to start with.

We can apply this technique to almost any area of life. "I will have two conversations with my spouse this week during which I listen without interrupting for at least five minutes." "I will limit my pretzel consumption to one a day, four days a week." There is nothing magical about a week; other time periods are okay. I try to have one or two action plans running most of the time. More than two at a time, though, is a setup for failure.

━ *Keep the Flow Going* ━

There are three more guidelines involved in the process of making change:

5. You will experience ups and downs. Drug and alcohol–abuse counselors tell me that most addicts have relapses. Good counselors often say to their clients in advance, "You will almost certainly backslide at some point. When you do, come back to me." Otherwise, when clients hit the inevitable bump in the road, they will feel like failures, bad people for whom there is no hope or help. Then it may be years before they quit again.

   The same rules apply to all kinds of behavior change. The great leap to fitness, the steadily improving ability to speak up for ourselves, or the sudden, permanent adoption of a healthy, natural diet—these things do not happen often. In real life there are good and bad days, good and bad weeks, months, even years. Coming back from the bad periods is part of the process.

   All kinds of changes and stresses can knock us off our program. We're walking every day, then we sprain an ankle. We're practicing daily relaxation when a noisy neighbor moves in and ruins the peace and quiet. Your partner leaves you, the rent goes up, you get bad news on a blood test, your child flunks out of college. Any of us could fill pages with similar things that have actually happened to us, and any of them can throw us for a loop. Good things can also throw us off schedule: a new job, a new love, an exciting cause or hobby. The important thing is to get back on track, because for each time we relapse and make a comeback we recover a little more quickly and easily.

6. Change takes longer than we think. It takes many weeks to lock in a new behavior. It's not like putting on a new pair of socks; it's more

like growing flowers in a plot already full of other plants. We have to tend to the new ones until they take hold. So be patient.

7. Change happens when we're not looking. We work and work toward getting in shape, say, or being more disciplined about finishing what we start. Nothing seems to happen for the longest time. Then one day we're rolling along in our wheelchair when we notice that we're not getting tired nearly as fast as we used to. We're breathing easier, feeling better. When did it happen? Most likely it happened when we stopped watching. When we give up the need for miracles is when miracles happen. And in the field of self-motivated behavior change, miracles happen every day.

◌ Habit Control

Changing behavior means changing habits, some of which, like substance abuse, are chronic conditions of their own. Smoking, for example, kills more people each year than cocaine, heroin, alcohol, marijuana, auto accidents, AIDS, murder, suicide, and fires combined. Americans spend millions each year trying to stop smoking, with spotty results. What accounts for the persistence of a habit so deadly, expensive, and outwardly unattractive? Yes, nicotine is addictive, but most smokers go through the pain of withdrawal repeatedly, only to start using again for reasons unrelated to physical dependency. The same pattern happens with other drugs and behaviors. If we really want to stop, why do we keep going?

What trips up most of us is our unquestioning belief that we "really want" to stop. It would be more accurate to say that part of us wants to stop. There is always another part that wants to continue the behavior; otherwise, we wouldn't. Part of us may be in rebellion against authority, may be lonely, may be in pain, may even want to die. We may relate smoking, drinking, or whatever to the feelings of comfort, support, or love we desperately need.

Psychologist Jonathan Diamond, who treats adolescent drug addicts, often has them write "good-bye letters" to their preferred drugs as a way of helping them uncover how they really feel about their addictions. The torrents of love, anger, need, pain, and loss in these letters reveal that

our relationships with habits are like relationships with people, places, or jobs. They are complex, painful, and difficult to break off.

It helps a lot when we become aware of the feelings behind our habits. Does smoking help us deal with a lack of love we felt in the past or present? Does drinking reduce our sense of guilt or frustration over our life situation? Writing a letter or keeping a journal can help us identify such negative or addictive patterns and habits. So can psychotherapy. Chapter 7 discusses the use of interactive guided imagery, a technique I use with clients.

When we are certain about our intention to change, we need a method and a source of support. Line up family and friends who will listen and do some handholding as necessary. Join a support group of some kind if that is appropriate. Identify things that trigger the behavior you are trying to change—certain people, places, activities, or feelings—and brainstorm ways to avoid those danger areas. In identifying triggers, remember the drug-treatment acronym H.A.L.T., which asks you to stop and identify if you're Hungry, Angry, Lonely, or Tired. Those are four pretty sure triggers.

Make a plan. For smoking cessation, you could choose "I will taper off cigarettes and stop within six weeks" or "I will quit now and use the patches as long as necessary." Break your larger goal down into action steps for each week. You could also ask your doctor about medication.

⌒Attitudes and Beliefs

Of all the amazing things I learned in researching this book, here is the most incredible: We can change our deepest thoughts, attitudes, and beliefs just by motivation and practice. This principle, the foundation of cognitive therapy, is a truly lifesaving proposition. Most of us wander around with thoughts and attitudes that damage our bodies and make us miserable, e.g., "I'm not good enough"; "My life has no meaning"; "People make me so angry"; "My mother didn't love me"; or "I can't get well." We can actually train ourselves to embrace healthier beliefs, which lead to healthier behaviors and healthier, happier lives. Clinicians around the country are carrying out such programs.

Dr. Naras Bhat, at Mount Diablo Hospital in California, runs a heart disease–reversal program with a high rate of success. To a plan of exercise,

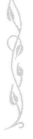

diet, social support, and relaxation, Dr. Bhat adds anger reduction. He motivates heart patients by having them think angry thoughts while hooked to a heart monitor and then showing them how their heart rate became more irregular and variable. He tells them, "The person you are angry with will still be walking around, and you will be dead of a heart attack."

Participants learn to monitor their emotional states and to disclose them to others. In fact, Bhat requires them to talk about their emotions every day to a significant other, because talking about the feelings and thoughts behind anger tends to defuse them. (If no one is available, the patient is matched with another program participant.) They deliberately replace thoughts like "That guy is an idiot" with new thoughts like "He's different, but he's not difficult." Then they practice the hell out of the new thoughts.

⸻ *Healthy and Unhealthy Beliefs* ⸻

Dr. Carl Simonton identifies five criteria for healthy beliefs, developed by cognitive psychologists. A healthy belief should do at least three of the following: be based on fact, protect our life and health, help us achieve short- and long-term goals, help us avoid undesirable conflicts, or help us feel the way we want to feel.

Dr. Simonton found that hopelessness and despair sharply limited his cancer patients' life expectancies. He noticed that these harmful feelings stemmed from unhealthy thoughts like "I can't get well" or "Nobody cares." Simonton's approach involves making people aware of the thoughts that are causing them pain (a classic cognitive-therapy strategy). The time to identify these thoughts is when we are in the unpleasant emotional state they cause. When we're anxious, panicky, angry, or depressed, those are the times to ask, "What am I thinking right now that is causing these feelings?" Simonton has patients write down their negative thoughts and apply the five tests for healthy beliefs. Then he works with them to develop positive alternatives.

For example, a depressed patient may be thinking, "I've never done anything worthwhile"—the kind of attitude that has been found to decrease survival time in cancer. But does this thought accord with the

facts? Does it help protect the patient's life and health, or help achieve short- and long-term goals? If patients can acknowledge an unhealthy belief, and if they are motivated (either by improved chances for survival or by a desire for less misery while alive), they can develop an alternative thought, such as "I do the best I can" or "People benefit from things I do" or even "The world is a better place because I am in it."

The new, positive statement must be something the person can believe, and he or she must practice saying it over and over to himself or herself. Some therapists have clients carry a list of their self-destructive beliefs and the healthier options. When one finds oneself carrying negative feelings, he or she takes out the list, identifies the recurrent damaging thought, and then recites to himself or herself the new, positive alternative. Amazingly, Dr. Bhat and Dr. Simonton both report that lasting change of belief, attitude, and behavior often happen in only three to six weeks! This is not too much work to change a lifetime of pain into a healthy outlook.

Take This Job, Please

Let's talk about changing other aspects of our lives that can cripple our health, starting with work—probably the number-one candidate for change. Few aspects of life bring as much pleasure and meaning to our lives as work, and few bring more pain and frustration. For most of us, work is our major interface with the outside world, a huge part of our identity; it is who we are, what we do. It is also our means of support, of maintaining a decent standard of living. We fear losing work; our earning power is crucial to our sense of self and our physical well-being.

Necessary as it is, work can injure us in a variety of ways. Working too many hours, changing shifts, or being exposed to environmental hazards can wear us down or make us sick. Work stations or tasks that encourage bad posture or repetitive-motion stress can lead to discomfort and illness.

More often, work damages us through psychosocial stress. I ask clients, "How is your relationship with your boss and your coworkers? Do you look forward to seeing them? Do you feel anxious or angry when thinking about going to work? Do you feel safe? Do you feel any sense of control over your job or your work environment?"

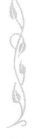

If answers to these questions are troubling, a change needs to be made. Feeling a lack of control at work has been strongly linked to immune system and cardiac problems. In fact, British studies have found that a low-ranking job with little power and many demands is a better predictor of early death than smoking, obesity, or high blood pressure.

The job of city bus operator involves the killer combination of high stress and low control, at least here in San Francisco. Operators have to meet impossible schedules over which they have no power, have to deal with unpredictable dangers such as unsafe auto drivers and pedestrians, and are subject to abuse from disgruntled passengers. Their schedules disallow exercise breaks and regular bathroom breaks. The design of seats and other equipment contributes to strain injuries.

Bus operators have extremely high rates of high blood pressure, diabetes, heart disease, and cancer. Poor health behaviors account for some of their elevated risk, but not nearly enough to explain their astronomical illness rates. And, their unhealthy behaviors, of course, also relate partly to their job. For example, few of us would feel like exercising after the kind of exhausting shift that they endure.

── *The Meaning of Our Work* ──

The meaning we find in our work also affects us deeply. Suppose two people deliver bottled water for a living. One might think, "This is great. I get out to different parts of the city, and I get to meet different people. I'm not stuck in an office or factory; I'm bringing people this good, healthy water. They're always happy to see me. I wish it paid more, but it beats welfare."

The other is thinking, "I hate this job. I could have been a lawyer if I hadn't dropped out of college. The company doesn't respect me; the managers never ask my opinion or let me plan my own routes. I can't raise a family on this pay. My back and feet hurt from lifting. The water is a rip-off; it's no better than tap water."

You wouldn't need to do a physical exam to suspect that the first worker is better off than her miserable counterpart. If our job holds positive meaning for us, then work can be a source of health as well as money. If the job seems a dead end or a detour, we may feel frustrated. If we work for a company or agency that does good work, we will tend to feel good about ourselves. If we can't find a way to believe our work is valuable, we may be at risk.

As with most parts of our lives, when it comes to changing work, we have three choices. We can leave, we can change the conditions of the job, or we can change the way we respond to it. Changing the conditions is hard; companies rarely alter the way they do business to meet the needs of one person. Cutting back to part-time or moving to another department might be possible, though, and the Americans with Disabilities Act might give us some leverage if we have a qualifying condition.

We can also change the way we respond physically. Most so-called repetitive strain injury is thought to be due to unrelieved tension and stress on the job rather than to any particular movements. Hundreds of millions of dollars are spent on changing workplace design when the real problem is supervisors who put extra stress on workers, and workers who don't breathe, stretch, or relax. We can prevent much work-related pain by taking frequent minibreaks, paying attention to our bodies' signals to relax tight muscles, and doing a lot of deep, focused breathing. Of course, some employers don't want us to do these things, wrongly believing they interfere with productivity, when in fact healthy work styles actually seem to improve production.

If other work-related dissatisfactions plague us, we can get creative about coming up with solutions. If the commute is stressful, we may be able to find a job closer to home or change our mode of transportation. Although some bosses are hard-liners, others may be willing to modify procedures if they are given a well thought-out reason. Better communication (addressed in Chapter 4) may resolve some unpleasantness with supervisors. Labor organizations are also a resource for those who have them.

⁓ *Knowing When to Quit* ⁓

Quitting or cutting back on work can bring about a crucial change in healing—in fact, I always encourage people to get out of abusive situations—but we might first want to have a plan for what to do next. Unemployment is more stressful than all but the worst jobs; however, with proper planning, job loss can usually be turned into a blessing. Do we need to take

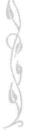

some classes, do some research, make some contacts, call in some favors? Are we willing to change careers completely? Perhaps there are things we have always wanted to do. A vocational counselor can help. We may want to look at getting needed training, finding potential employers, getting a résumé together, or figuring out how to make our finances work.

We may be able to work on a contractual basis, which is more flexible than hourly. We may be able to start our own business or job share. In looking for a new job, we may want to check into flexibility of hours, opportunities for restful breaks, and convenience of bathroom use. The issue of whether to tell prospective employers about an illness has no simple solution; it's case by case. I've found, though, that work relationships are less comfortable when coworkers think you're hiding something from them, even if it is, strictly speaking, none of their business.

Often, the very fact that we know we are working our way out of an unpleasant situation makes the situation more tolerable. The possibility of being without work for an extended period is a very scary prospect. But if we are going to be too sick to work anyway, what's the good of hanging on to something that may be killing us?

That said, it might be worthwhile first to try identifying and changing an attitude or behavior. Practice relaxing and breathing more, or search for the value in what the company does. Talk with satisfied coworkers or customers to find out what they like about the company. Unpleasant or threatening relationships with superiors can be much harder matters to reframe. Sometimes we can learn to see things from their perspective, which may make it easier to let go of resentment and to stay on their good side.

People with major illness often have fewer work choices because of disability, decreased stamina, or the effects of medical treatment. Some may have to cope with long-term—even permanent—unemployment. It helps to remember that there is a difference between a job and work. We can perform very valuable work even if we can't physically participate in a full-time job. Additionally, disability insurance and social security are available as sources of financial support (see Chapter 4); as little as they pay, people can still enjoy good lives with those forms of income.

Relationships

Relationships, especially committed partnerships such as marriage, can cause even more pain and bring even more healing than work does. In particular, feeling unloved or as though we have nobody to love puts a damper on our appreciation of life. Or, if we have to tiptoe around our partner or another family member, if every interaction with him or her is a source of conflict, threat, or annoyance, life can seem more trouble than it's worth. On the other hand, a loving, supportive relationship can sustain us through trials we never thought we could survive.

When we contract a significant illness—or preferably before that point—we frequently need to change something about our pattern of connection with one or more important people in our lives. Again, we have the choice of separating from the relationship, changing it, or changing our response to it.

Recovery literature abounds with stories of people who healed in near-miraculous fashion after a relationship change. Sometimes people recover from terminal cancer after divorce from or death of an abusive spouse. Others, apparently at death's door, have healed when they found new loves (Chapter 5). Still others have far outlived their prognoses after children or grandchildren came into their lives.

Usually, the question is not one of dumping someone or of finding someone new, but of improving the love relationships we have. The key usually lies in better communication, a topic covered extensively in Chapter 4. Sometimes we have to care for family members with severe illness or disability, which can be extremely stressful for the caregivers. Here the key lies in getting help. Improving relationships with other family members and close friends also pays off. If these relationships can't be improved, we may need to let them go. If you find yourself exhausted every time a particular friend visits, maybe he or she should visit somebody else.

Places of Refuge

When we think of home, we like to envision a place of love and support—or at least one that smells good. Often, though, our houses or apartments, which should be healing, can make us sick. The environment may be laden

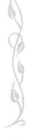

with chemicals, molds, or dirt, provoking asthma or respiratory infections. Noise levels can keep us awake and on edge, raising our blood pressure. There may be fighting words flying around inside the house and bullets flying around outside, or the place may be disorderly or ugly, lacking any touch of nature to lighten our spirits. Living in such stressful, unsafe situations makes staying healthy much more difficult.

As with our jobs and our relationships, we can change our environment, change our reaction to it, or leave. Changing the environment might involve planting gardens, getting rid of rugs or drapes that hold dust, cleaning with nontoxic soaps, sweeping the streets, or getting involved with a neighborhood organization to beautify the area or to address unsafe conditions, to name just a few possibilities.

Changing our reaction to our living environment involves practicing coping mechanisms. I lived two blocks from a hospital and three blocks from a fire station for fifteen years. There was no way to stop the sirens that screamed day and night. Earplugs and tape players with earphones got me to sleep. Obviously, if we feel unsafe walking past a particular corner in the neighborhood, we should look for other routes; they almost always exist.

One of the best ways to improve a living situation is to make more friends in the area. There may be some beautiful people we haven't taken the time to get to know. There may be some great sources of help or of ideas for coping. Friends can make a neighborhood a home.

The third option, finding a new place to live, frequently involves financial hardships or sacrifices. It may take planning, saving, and a lot of work. It may require reaching out to friends and other sources of help. It may mean giving up other things. It is not a decision taken lightly, but it can make a huge difference in our lives and health.

While we are in the process of changing work or home situations, or if such changes are not possible immediately, we can still determine to take the best possible care of ourselves in other ways. By exercising, relaxing, enjoying life more fully, and generally caring for our minds, bodies, and spirits, we can often fight off some of the negative effects of harmful situations.

⌐A Continuous Process

One successful change leads to another, and in the process we begin to feel more and more in control. Life can get better and better—if only because many of us start from pretty low places. The process never really stops; we can always feel better, find more well-being.

Laura George, a fifty-three-year-old with hypertension, told me that since being diagnosed at age forty-one, she has changed work twice in an attempt to find something more fulfilling and less stressful. She also has started yoga, moved to a quieter neighborhood, educated herself about her condition, gone back to school, and started working out, in addition to taking prescribed medicines and monitoring her blood pressure.

She says all these changes have helped. Her life is better than ever, and she is on the lookout for more things she can do to become a better, healthier person. She currently works part-time, is active in her church, takes care of her family, and watches the neighbors' kids two days a week. What an interesting life! She couldn't do it, though, without a number of sources of support. We all need help, which is the subject of the next chapter.

ALL THE HELP
WE CAN GET

If someone doesn't need help or support in some way,
they're not living right.

AIDS survivor Oscar Stiebel

THEY SAY THREE STRIKES AND YOU'RE OUT, but when Sharon walked into Project Eve, my mother's training program for displaced homemakers in Buffalo, New York, she already had at least six strikes against her. At thirty-three, she lacked even a high school education. She had a troubled adolescent son, an abusive husband, and a drinking problem. Her only recent paying job was prostitution, which doesn't carry much weight on a résumé. And one other thing—she had cancer. Doctors recommended surgery, radiation, and chemotherapy, offering a fifty-fifty chance of five-year survival, with treatment.

Like most victims of domestic violence, Sharon was isolated, and she had been for a long time. Her parents had ignored her; her husband kept her alone and fearful. The women in the Project Eve program became her support system. They encouraged and protected her through divorcing her man and through chemotherapy. They pushed her to go back to school and to stop drinking.

Incredibly, twenty years later, Sharon is now a lawyer with a successful career, a good love relationship, and no evidence of cancer. Who or what gets credit for this amazing change? Her own inner resources, her doctors, and her teachers certainly played roles, but she says the most important thing was the support of the Project Eve women. With them, she finally experienced connection.

Support makes the difference. With enough help—human, spiritual, and/or financial—people can overcome situations that seem worse than hopeless. Without support, fully manageable conditions may spiral out of control and destroy our quality of life or kill us prematurely. The importance of social support for health has been documented in over thirty studies in various countries. Every kind of health problem occurs more often and with more damaging effects among those who are isolated.

Of course, we would all have more social support if we could. Unfortunately, many of us face powerful social and psychological barriers against forming new connections and even stronger ones against seeking help from the people we already know. This chapter shows where these barriers come from and suggests ways around them. It teaches how to find potential sources of support, strengthen our relationships, ask for and accept help, and build a support system. Particular attention is paid to getting the best results from our health-care team. The chapter devotes much attention to improving communication, especially assertiveness, which is usually key to better relationships.

Isolation Epidemic

It is frightening how little support some people have and how much difficulty some have asking for help. In my work as a telephone triage nurse, I would often advise patients in mild distress—well enough to walk but not to drive—to come to the emergency room, only to have them reply they had no one to bring them. A conversation similar to the following would ensue:

Me: No one? Nobody at all?

Caller: Nope. (Cough.) I don't have anybody.

Me: A friend? A relative? A neighbor? Someone from your church, maybe?

Caller: Well, my friends are dead. And I don't really know the people around here. I've only been here five years. (Groan.) Can't I get an ambulance?

Me: What about your children? Or grandchildren?

Caller: My children are all out of state. Except Sheila. And she's ninety minutes away, and she has to go to work in the morning. I couldn't call her.

We then have to decide whether to order an ambulance, which is probably needed for more urgent cases, and whose bill the health-insurance plan and the caller would fight over for the next six years. When we become so removed from human support that we have nobody we are willing or able to call, even in a life-threatening situation, how can we expect to stay well?

Unfortunately, isolation is built into American culture and increasingly into global culture. People change jobs, homes, and cities repeatedly. The primary American social unit, the nuclear family, leaves many of us emotionally and physically distant from aunts, cousins, grandparents, or grandchildren who might otherwise help. Our social mobility and emphasis on independence may also keep us from getting to know our neighbors, who are the most geographically suited to provide friendship and support.

Social connection means more than just a source of transportation. We all need to feel connected to the larger world; otherwise, why are we here? I know several elders whose recurrent health problems, necessitating frequent hospital visits, sharply improved when they started getting regular visits from family and friends. People with chronic illness often need help with the work of self-maintenance, such as cooking, shopping, and housework. If we don't get it, we wind up eating poorly or suffering other health-damaging problems. The solution is to ask for help, but many, for reasons explained in this chapter, find that very hard to do.

☞ The John Wayne Syndrome

Cheri Register interviewed dozens of people, mostly women, for her book *The Chronic Illness Experience*. She found that most were reluctant to "bother" people. It seemed many felt "unworthy" of special attention. She quotes one woman as saying, "Asking for help is, first off, an admission of helplessness.... It certainly seems un-American." Other women told Register they feared becoming "burdensome."

These feelings are natural in a society where independence is the virtue most highly prized, the thing we strive for from the age of two, the quality our male movie heroes exemplify as they ride across the screen on horses, in sports cars, or aboard jets. Even female cultural figures now embody a fierce independence most of the time. Yet modern society is more interdependent than any before. Probably hundreds of people (plus animals and plants) were involved in producing and getting to you the food you ate yesterday. In point of fact, we do not live, progress, succeed, or fail as individuals, but as aggregates: families, teams, companies, communities. Nobody makes it on their own, but many of us die that way, because we are too isolated. We don't know how to ask for assistance.

There are other barriers to seeking help. Neuropsychologist Darcy Cox, who works with and studies people with chronic illness, says people often don't ask for help because they are afraid of rejection or dependence. She says, "It makes some people very angry when they have to ask for help. When people get sick, asking for help is an admission that they really are sick. Asking for help, for a lot of people, feels like a defeat. When it reaches the point where they have to ask for help, it sometimes feels like the disease has won."

When Pneumocystis carinii pneumonia hit Rob Mitchell's AIDS-weakened body, he had to choose between independence and life. "A life-giving decision," he says, "was to accept help when I needed it. I probably would not be alive today if I hadn't gotten over that, if I hadn't learned that it's okay to call Mom and Dad and say, 'I don't want to go into the hospital. Will you come and take care of me?'"

In spite of the high stakes, most of us find asking for help a difficult and painful thing to do. My friend Elaine fought like a demon against becoming dependent because of her MS. Reliant on a wheelchair for

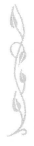

mobility, she still did most of the housework and cooking. Her loving husband would offer help, and she hated it. She fought him off, insisting on doing more than she comfortably could, refusing to use her limited energy for healing. As a result, she frequently wound up on the floor, needing assistance from the fire department or neighbors to get her back into bed. She ended up even more dependent because her MS worsened rapidly from the stress.

—— *"I Hate to Ask"* ——

Here are several reasons people cite for not getting help, with some of the arguments I use to help clients overcome them:

1. **"People don't like to help." ("They're too busy." "They will be annoyed.")**

   Actually, most people like to help. It makes them feel good. Yes, there are occasional jerks. When I get on a crowded bus, some people will offer a seat, while some won't even move their packages off the seat next to them. In general, though, it's heartwarming how willingly people help; it makes me feel we belong to a pretty decent species.

2. **"I will feel like a burden."**

   Ask yourself something like, "If the roles were reversed, would I want her to ask me? How would I feel about helping her? Would I think she was being a burden?" I remind clients that we've all helped a lot of people in our time and that by not asking, they are depriving their friends of opportunities to feel good about themselves. We may have to address the hidden self-esteem issue here: the thought that "I am not worthy of being helped."

3. **"I don't like to be dependent."**

   Well, maybe nobody likes it, but we are all dependent on each other, all the time (as I mentioned above, think about all the people, plants, and animals involved in bringing you your last meal or in making the furniture you're sitting on this very minute). Interdependence

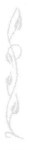

is how life works. We've been sold a fantasy of independence and freedom mainly designed to encourage us to buy more. Real freedom depends on having others on whom we can rely.

4. **"If people help me, I will owe them." (This one is often unspoken.)**

We will owe them, although they probably won't care. They owe others, just as others owe us. If we want to pay them back, though, our gratitude, love, and friendship will go a long way. We can also do things within our power for those who help us, or we can do for others even less fortunate.

Cheri Register says such networks of caring and helping were characteristic of her small-town childhood environment:

> Growing up in a small town taught me that mutual caring is not just a one-to-one matter. It is a communal activity. When the course of someone's life is drastically altered . . . the neighbors know just what to do. They bring food: hot dishes, cakes, vegetables, or bowls of jello. There is no obligation to refill the bowl [before returning it to its owner], though some people do. . . . It is simply understood that, over the years, everyone will give and receive their fair share.

In other words, not only are other people part of our team, we are part of theirs.

Build a Network

Everyone needs help, and those of us with major health problems may need more help than others do. It's a bad idea to get it all in one place—from a spouse, for instance. We'll just burn out the caregiver and miss out on other, potentially more effective, help. Nobody is good at everything. For example, we may need someone to help us shop, cook, or do housework or someone to give us a break with the children or elders in our care. We may want someone to go with us to doctor appointments or someone

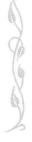

to listen to our feelings or to help us sort out our treatment options. We probably will want to talk with people who are going through the same problems we have. We may even want someone to push us to do more self-care or maybe someone to exercise with us. Obviously, one person cannot do all these things.

If we are confined to our home for lengthy periods, we may want visitors and phone calls to keep us in touch with the world. We may benefit by being prayed for. We may need someone to touch us, hold our hand, or to fight for us when we are helpless in the hospital. We may need personal care. Possibly we will need to ask for money. Whatever our state of health, we need some kind of support network.

Where is all this help going to come from? Ideally, we have a group including family, friends, neighbors, health professionals, possibly volunteers, and, if necessary, social agencies. Usually family members are the first people we turn to for help. We don't want to impose on them, we don't necessarily want them to see us "at our worst," but in most cases they will help, if asked. Don't stop there, though; try to line up a large network of helpers. That way, we get to spend time with a whole variety of people, we avoid overtaxing any one source, and we probably get more done.

⟶ *The Right Friend for the Job* ⟵

Register recommends finding the right friends for various needs. Some may be great at housework, but lousy listeners. Some may be good advocates, but not want to touch you or do any personal care. Not everyone is going to want or be able to do the intense stuff. Oscar Stiebel remembers friends who, when he was terribly ill, "thought they were really taking care of me, when all they were doing was calling once in a while, and I was too tired to talk anyway." (That kind of help is often important, though.)

More intimate friends may want to do more intimate things—then again they may not—while more casual friends may help with things like shopping. We often worry that we will drive friends away, and that is possible if we overuse them. Most of the time, though, helping actually deepens a friendship, according to Register and other authorities.

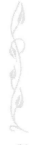

⟶ *Religious and Voluntary Organizations* ⟵

When my friend Beth's chronic fatigue was at its worst, members of her church came by with food and helped with housework. My coworker Ella had church members at her bedside constantly when she was hospitalized for pancreatic cancer, and she lived for eighteen months after her diagnosis—more than three times the five-month average. Church groups are often excellent resources for that kind of support. They'll also pray for us, and prayer possesses documented, though disputed, power to help us get well. Not that a dying person will jump out of bed and go running down the hall in response to prayer. Those types of miracles are exceedingly rare, but highly significant improvement following prayer or other kinds of so-called "distance healing" has been shown in patients with heart disease and AIDS. Researchers are currently studying prayer's efficacy in other conditions.

Disease-specific organizations like the Cancer Society and the Arthritis Foundation or service organizations such as the Kiwanis Club can also be sources of help. Church-related groups like Catholic Social Services often help people of all religions. We need to look around—in the phone book, at the library, on the Internet, in the hospital social-work department, or in the resource lists at the back of books like this one.

⟶ *Support Groups* ⟵

Support groups exist for almost any conceivable shared situation, from alcoholism to cancer to divorce to unemployment. This is a good thing, because as our life situations change we often need to be around new people who can relate to our new challenges and problems. If we are quitting smoking, for example, we probably need to be around others who are trying to quit—and we may also need some new nonsmoking friends after we quit. Old friends, as Oscar found out, can't always deal with our new conditions.

Psychologist Joan Klagsbrun, of Watertown, Massachusetts, sets up support groups for people dealing with major health problems. She says these groups can have a powerful effect on the course of illness and the death rates of participants. In one study, support groups that met ninety minutes a week for six weeks were found to make cancer patients less

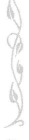

depressed, more vigorous, and better able to handle their feelings. Their immune systems also functioned better, and five to six years after the support groups ended participants had died at only one-third the rate of the control group!

Some of the participants probably kept in touch with each other after the group ended, thus receiving ongoing support. Support groups are a good way to meet people. Some are "closed" groups, where people sign up for a set period of time and, it is hoped, bond with each other. Others are "drop-in" groups, allowing participants to come and go as they please. Drop-in groups form less solid connections, but they expose participants to greater numbers of people. All support groups are sources of information. Some also include visualization, relaxation, or emotional-processing exercises.

One problem with disease-specific support groups is that we may have little in common with the other participants except a shared diagnosis. We may not feel like socializing or making friends in such a group, but we can learn from fellow participants that we are not alone, and we can obtain good information. Fortunately, a number of groups are usually available, at least in urban areas, and at least one of them should be suitable for your needs. Classes and lectures related to your condition (such as those offered by the HL groups I work with) can also serve as a support group, bringing people together who share similar situations.

Support groups might feel frightening or intimidating. People may attend who are much sicker than we are or who appear to be dying or severely disabled. We may not want to be confronted with the thought that their condition could happen to us. Some people also find themselves bored with listening to others talk about their illness-related problems meeting after meeting. If it's a drop-in group, we can simply attend when we feel like it and skip when we don't.

— *Parents and Other Family* —

Getting help from parents, siblings, and children can bring up hard emotional issues. We may have spent twenty years or more becoming independent of our parents. How can we return to their care? If our parents are elderly, we may feel we should be taking care of them or at least allowing them to enjoy their retirement.

Conversely, we have always taken care of our children, and it seems wrong for them to have to take care of us. But adult children as well as younger kids can benefit from taking on more responsibility. Even when children live at home, we often don't ask them to pull their weight, a pattern that leaves them without the necessary skills to take care of themselves or of anyone else.

Our relationships with siblings, parents, or children may be strained or distant. We may have to let go of some old resentments and hurts if we and our families are to tolerate or thrive in a closer relationship. A relative who always criticized us when we were healthy is unlikely to ease up just because we are sick. We may have to learn better ways of communicating with a helper who gives us more stress than support, or we may have to choose between letting go of being hurt by their attitude or deciding that their support isn't worth the trouble. Still, helping and being helped by family members can strengthen our sense of self by healing our connections.

"It was rough having my parents come to take care of me," Rob Mitchell told me. "Particularly difficult was seeing how stressed out and at a loss to handle it my father was. My mother had already taken care of my late partner, Rick, and my sister's husband, Ron, when they had pneumocystis, and they had both died. So my parents knew the practical aspects. In the end, having them in my house and helping out turned out to be a source of strength and comfort for me. Having my parents there in the house with me, I felt safe again."

Rather than focusing on our increased dependence, we should emphasize the renewal and deepening of our family ties. In this way, health problems can be opportunities for the whole family to become closer. This will usually depend upon improved communication, which we'll discuss shortly. Usually we can help family members improve their behavior at the same time we learn to deal with them better.

⟶ *Home-Care Workers* ⟵

Sometimes the best available help is hired help. Luis Calderon, of Consumers in Action for Personal Assistance, says people often refuse home-care assistance, even when it's paid for by insurance. "Many people have no experience being an employer, supervising someone," he says. "Or they're afraid to let a stranger into their home. So they wind up hurting themselves in falls or cooking accidents, or they spend all their time and energy doing housework that someone else could easily do, when they could be in the park or visiting friends." Excellent nonprofit and for-profit home-care agencies exist in most cities. Do some research, ask around, and hire someone, if appropriate.

❧ *Health Professionals* ❧

We obviously want to find the best possible network of health professionals, including doctors, nurses, therapists, alternative healers, whoever. The best ones are not always those with the biggest reputations or the fanciest offices. Even more important may be how they communicate with us, and we with them.

It's important to remember that the healer is sometimes as important as the method. Dr. Bernie Siegel says a good doctor will demonstrate compassion, acceptance, availability, openness with information, a sense of humor, and the ability to accept criticism. That's a tall order, but we want those qualities. On the other hand, if we're facing a difficult surgery or a complicated treatment, we might opt, just for that one procedure, to use a super-specialist who also happens to be a jerk. Usually, whether we are considering a top-flight medical/surgical specialist or a street-corner herbalist, we want to find someone we like and who seems to like us.

There are some kinds of healers we don't want. When cyclist Lance Armstrong was seeking a second opinion on chemotherapy for his metastatic cancer, he went to a hotshot specialist at a university hospital in Texas. This doctor told him, "Every day I'm going to kill you, then bring you back to life. You are going to crawl out of here. . . . You will never ride your bike again." The specialist said any other approach would leave Armstrong dead. Maybe some patients would have found this approach encouraging, but most of us, I venture, would be terrified. Fortunately, with the support of his family Lance walked out and got a third opinion from a less extreme, more caring team at the University of Indiana, who helped save his life and his career. Eventually he inspired millions by winning the Tour de France, the world's biggest bicycle race, three years in a row.

Siegel describes other doctors to avoid. He tells of a man with a sign on his desk reading, "Compromise means doing it my way"; another who didn't want his patients to read any books on their condition; and a physician who when challenged by a patient yelled, "There will be only one f___ing cook in this kitchen." We should refuse to settle for behavior like this from doctors or other healers—unless we make a conscious decision that that particular doctor or healer is the best person for a specific aspect of our care. Even then we should remember that *we* are in charge, even if the doctor doesn't believe it.

Here's one other piece of advice: If you sign up to participate in a research study, don't use the researcher as your primary doctor. Research tends to divide loyalties between the success of the study and the welfare of the patient. You need a doctor who is looking out for you, not thinking about the quality of his or her experimental data.

⌒ Get the Most from Your Healers

Doctors tend to be overworked and frequently frustrated by their inability to be the healing gods everyone expects. It's hard for them, as it is for us, when they can't cure us or even reduce our symptoms. They are trained to be fixers, not coaches helping us to do for ourselves. Few medical schools do a decent job of teaching medical students to communicate with or motivate their patients. As a result of our doctor worship, many patients don't speak up, and many doctors don't listen. The result can be suboptimal treatment and, often, dangerous mistreatment. Medical error, in fact, is the eighth leading cause of death in the United States, according to a 1999 report from the Institute of Medicine.

We need to be assertive with health professionals. Without getting angry, tell the doctor, "I didn't understand that explanation. Why am I taking this medication?" Or, "This diet list you gave me doesn't have any foods I like on it. Please connect me with someone who can provide more ideas." Don't accept put-downs or reassurances that fail to ring true. I've even heard of people being assertive in ambulances, as in, "Please turn off that siren; it's making me really scared. You're taking good care of me; I'll be okay until we get to the hospital."

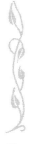

Patients often have lots of questions and little time with the doctor. We should prepare a written list of concerns and questions, with the most important ones first. Read from the list or give it to him or her, along with our report on how we are doing (see Chapter 6). The doctor probably won't have time to answer ten questions, but he or she can answer the first two or three and may be willing to look at the rest later and to answer them by phone or mail or at the next appointment. Unfortunately, as patients, we are often too stressed in the doctor's office to take in everything. I recommend tape recording your consultation with the doctor and listening to it at home or bringing someone along to take notes.

Ken Wong, who has probably led more HL classes than anyone else, has several suggestions for getting the most from doctors. He tries to book the first morning appointment or the first appointment after lunch so he gets seen before the doctor gets backed up.

"I always try to identify with the doctor as a person," Ken says. "If there are pictures of his family in the office, I ask about them. If he has children around my son's age, I ask about their schools and tell him about my son's. It helps him think of me as a person, not just a patient." Doctors need love too. A handshake and some words of thanks will definitely make the doctor's day and encourage him or her to see us as real people.

⸻ *Bring Your Team with You* ⸻

Unless we are exceptionally good at asserting ourselves, we may want to bring an advocate with us to doctor appointments. A friend or family member provides another set of eyes and ears and may remember things later that we have forgotten because of stress. People who care about us are much more likely to speak up for us than we are for ourselves. It's amazing how militant some people can get about protecting others, when the same loudmouths would just let the system roll over them without a word of protest if they were the patient.

It's especially important to have advocates when we're in the hospital, because the risks are higher and our ability to speak for ourselves is often limited. For Ken Wong, his wife acts as guardian. "When I was at Doctor's Hospital," he recalls, "I would have been walked all over by people because I was kind of dazed, out of it. One time I was bleeding after an angiogram; she spoke up for me to the doctors and nurses."

In the hospital it is best to have someone with us at all times (someone who knows how to be quiet when we need to rest). It's a good idea to have some tasty food brought in and maybe some comfort items such as pictures or a favorite blanket. Most importantly, we need advocates to protect us by, say, getting us moved if our roommate is noisy or by questioning a nurse who comes in to do an unexpected procedure or to give us a new and unexplained medicine.

Let's Talk About It

Many times the support we need is available. The problem is getting on the same page with our loved ones and the rest of our potential team. Marian came to HL class complaining about her husband, Tom. He made fun of her plans for exercise and opposed her efforts to eat healthier food. At least, that's what she told us. When he came in for a session, he actually sounded pretty supportive. The problem was communication: Marian hadn't really told him what she wanted and why. She had just kind of hinted at it and expected him to understand. After thirty-five years of talking past each other, they both assumed the other would oppose them; it had been years since either of them had even asked the other for what they wanted.

We have to do better than that. If we have a spouse or significant other, he or she will usually be the most important connection in our lives. The quality of that relationship has more effect on our health than almost anything else, and that quality depends on the quality of our communication. Come to think of it, the quality of all our relationships depends on good communication. Too often, we expect our loved ones to be mind readers. We get mad at them for not meeting our needs when we have never clearly told them what our needs or preferences are.

There are lots of reasons communication breaks down. Thousands of psychotherapists make good livings doing little besides helping families improve their communication patterns. Communication skills are not rocket science, though. They really come down to three habits anyone can learn: assertiveness, listening, and emotional disclosure.

～ *Assertiveness* ～

Assertiveness means clearly stating what we need, want, or believe, without infringing on the rights of others. For example, "I would love to hear about your day, honey, but I am doing my relaxation now. Would thirty minutes from now be all right?" Or, "I know you like to smoke, but it bothers my lungs. Please do it outside the house."

Assertiveness means standing up for ourselves, and doing so can be scary at first. Many of us have learned to suppress our wants and needs, to just go along, and sometimes that is appropriate. But most often we deny ourselves needed care for reasons that don't actually make sense. Psychologist Albert Ellis points out that we often believe that if we assert ourselves, others will get mad and their anger will destroy us. We believe that saying "no" will hurt others and that their pain will be our fault, or we think it's wrong to deny others' requests, even if our own needs are greater. In practice, though, the sky does not fall when we speak up for ourselves; most often, people will respect us more when we respect ourselves.

Assertive communication consists mostly of "I" messages, that is, saying what "I" think, feel, and want, as opposed to focusing on what "you" have done wrong or how bad "you" are. For example, "I am frustrated that you didn't bring the car back when you said you would, because I was late for my appointment. I hate being late, and I was really stressed out. I'm angry that you didn't at least call me."

Note how much more constructive this sounds than using blame-filled "you" statements like the following: "You really messed me up! How could you lie about bringing the car back when you knew I needed it? You ruined my whole day, just like you always do!"

Both messages address the same problems, but which version will get a better response? The listener hears the "you" message as an attack and feels forced to defend himself or herself, and the two people end up farther apart. By contrast, the "I" message allows the listener to understand what the speaker is going through, and then he or she can work on fixing the problem rather than fighting back. It is never helpful to attack a person we care about; instead, we want to limit our criticism to a particular behavior that hurt us while assuring the other person that we still value him or her.

The basic form of the "I" message is as follows: "I feel X, when you do Y" (or "when this happens"), because it affects me in such and such a way." "I" messages are valuable because they force us to put into words what we are feeling. Until we have to say what we feel, we may not know what it is. Often we feel only anger and resentment, which are usually reactions to other painful feelings such as hurt or fear or feeling ignored, frustrated, or disrespected. By formulating our emotions into words, we clarify them for the other person and for ourselves. When we understand our own motivation we will be less likely to feel guilty for asking for more consideration.

Assertiveness isn't just for the hard stuff. An easier form of assertiveness involves giving sincere compliments and appreciation when warranted. "I really feel good that you bought my favorite kind of cereal." "You really look good in that outfit." Compliments and thanks shouldn't be faked—most people can spot insincerity—but honest compliments benefit both the giver and the recipient.

Assertiveness takes practice. We may be in the habit of saying "yes" to any request without first taking the time to think about and decide whether it is something we really can do and want to do. Then we feel stressed and angry about doing the thing we should have refused. We can avoid getting overcommitted in the first place by not rushing to respond to a request. Say, "I'll get back to you" or "Give me a day to think about it." We don't have to say "yes" automatically. Personal coach Cheryl Richardson says to give yourself extra time: "If you think a project will take you one week, say it will take two.... When you're asked what time you can make a meeting or a date, add extra time." Instead of booking yourself into a permanent rush, take time to think about what really works for you, and assert yourself accordingly.

— Disclosure —

Honestly disclosing our feelings has its own health benefits: Speaking our emotions removes a big source of stress. Feeling understood by those close to us enables us to relax and feel better. Honesty and disclosure can carry the risk of rejection or criticism, though, so we often shy away from them. Many cultures discourage talking about emotions, perhaps because they

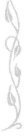

can seem disruptive of order and structure in a household or community. (If done well, though, sharing feelings tends to deepen connection and commitment.)

We need to learn the vocabulary of feelings before we can talk about them, and children, especially boys, often are not taught names for emotions, which leaves them no way to express feelings except by acting out. We reach adulthood without the experience of having emotions respected and addressed. This is unfortunate, because as Daniel Goleman points out in his book *Emotional Intelligence*, knowing about emotions can be more valuable than anything learned from books. People who are aware of their emotions and know how to deal with them have a big advantage.

Like assertiveness, disclosure takes practice. At first it may seem strange or wimpy to say, "I feel hurt," instead of, "You jerk!" We may find it hard to say, "I'm scared of what will happen if my condition gets any worse," so we just worry silently instead. Each time we open up, though, we will likely find that doing so brings us closer to our loved ones. Plus, sharing at this level gets easier with time. Of course, our loved ones don't always want to hear about our emotions, or vice versa, so we sometimes have to be willing to put the discussion off until later.

Active Listening

Perhaps more important than *what* we say is how well we listen. Many people, in or out of relationships, feel chronically unheard. Many of us tend to answer someone speaking to us before we've really heard what they had to say. We tend to jump in with our side of the story or our proposed solution when what the other person really wants is to be heard. If we improve our listening skills, our relationships usually improve wonderfully—and people will think we are really cool. Unlike assertiveness and disclosure, active listening isn't scary and can't cause arguments. Listening is one way people with chronic conditions can give something back to those who help us.

Here are some basic listening techniques:

Breathing—Taking some deep breaths will help keep us from interrupting the other person.

Silence—Simply sitting there as the other person talks will seem very supportive, although we may need to use gestures, such as moving a little closer or nodding, to indicate we're still paying attention.

Verbal encouragers—"Mm-hmm," "Uh-huh," "Go on," "Say a little more about that," and other such phrases may help a person come out with what they need to say.

Repeating—Simply repeating what the other person has said will let them know they have been heard and will encourage them to expand on it. At first this technique can feel strange, but usually it is a powerful response, especially if the speaker has said something with strong emotion.

Paraphrasing—Mirroring what the speaker tells you, but in your own words, indicates that you have understood them. It may also help them hear for themselves what they are actually saying. Your spouse says, "I can't stand my job." You could paraphrase, "Your job is really hard for you right now." Or you could go one step farther and use reflective listening, which involves mirroring back not only the words but also the emotions behind the words, e.g., "It sounds like you're really feeling frustrated with your work right now." Often, the feelings people express are more important to them than the facts of their case.

☞ More Tips for Better Love

Communication isn't the whole answer to better intimate relationships, though it goes a long way. It's also important to have boundaries, a place where other people stop and you start. We need to be able to separate and come closer as needed. Psychologist Darcy Cox says we need to be willing to do things on our own when possible: "We need to be able to say things like, 'I really want to do this, and if you don't want to do it, I hear that, but I'm going to do it anyway.' You have to take responsibility for getting your own needs met. If you want to see a movie, and the person you usually see movies with doesn't like that movie and won't go, . . . you have to take responsibility for going to see it. It's not their fault if you don't go see it."

If we refuse to do things without our partners, we put way too much pressure on them. We'll wear them out. And if we never learn to say "no," we'll wear ourselves out. If we have health problems, we have to remember that our partners have problems, too. They worry about us, and they wonder what the future holds, just like we do. Too often, these crucial topics are never discussed.

> Leah, a young medical student, developed a rare connective-tissue disease that has made it increasingly difficult to walk. She says it was harder for her husband David than for her: His concept of what his life was going to be included things like going on long bike rides through other parts of the world, seeing a lot of things on foot or by bike or whatever, doing those things with his life partner. So he had to give up a lot of his concepts of his own life, in the absence of any physical limitations on his part at all. That was very difficult. It was also difficult for me to relate to how difficult it was for him.

This was a hard transition for Leah and David. They went to couples therapy, which helped, and they gradually realized they could still do things together. When David went skiing, Leah stayed in the lodge, having a good time and communicating with him by walkie-talkie. They may go on a road trip through Europe—he on a bike, she on a motorized scooter.

Beth's chronic fatigue, at its worst, put a great strain on her relationship. Her reluctance to slow down left her without energy for her partner. She would say, "I have to get this work done, and then we'll sit and talk." Finally, she says, she "had to realize that that doesn't work, because if I am limited, he deserves a fair share of whatever energy I've got, even if it's not a lot." Like Leah and David's, Beth's improved marriage developed from improved communication.

☙ How to Ask for Help

My nurse friend Lindsay had never asked for help in her adult life, and lupus wasn't going to make her start. "What I would do," she remembers, "is push myself until I collapsed, and then they *had* to take care of me." Needless to say this is an inefficient method of getting help.

A general rule to follow when asking for help is to ask simply and specifically, without apologies. Just say, "Could you please carry this bag for me?" or "Please help me open this bottle." The guidebook *Living a Healthy Life with Chronic Conditions* cautions against vague requests, such as, "Could you help me move this weekend?" Favors that sound open-ended can scare people off. Be specific. "I have about six boxes of books I would like to move Saturday. It will probably take about an hour." People will be glad to do almost anything if they know what's involved so they can plan accordingly.

As Cheri Register's friend Peggy Evans points out, "I'm free to ask for help if they're free to say no." That's a good thing to let our potential helpers know; otherwise, we'll be afraid we're imposing on unwilling friends. Reinforce the point occasionally.

Of course, we want to remember to give thanks to our helpers—and also reassurance, if possible. Cancer survivor Lance Armstrong writes:

> One thing you realize when you're sick is that you aren't the only person who needs support—sometimes you have to be the one who supports others. My friends shouldn't always have to be the ones saying, "You're going to make it." Sometimes I had to be the one who reassured them, "I'm going to make it. Don't worry."

⌒ Social Services

With apologies to my social-worker friends, nobody wants a case manager or a social worker. Needing one makes us feel incompetent. Sometimes, though, government agencies can help with money, paying for medicines, finding housing, bringing in meals or household help, even supplying fuel oil or firewood for the winter.

My friend Oscar Stiebel has become an expert on obtaining benefits through the system. "A lot of times," he says, "the agencies want to help, but they're blocked by regulations. You have to help them help you." To qualify for firewood, Oscar has listed his dog as a dependent. He has fudged his address to be included in a geographically based program. "The way I look at it," he says, "they wanted me to have the benefit. So my getting evicted and having to leave the city—it's best they don't know about that. You have to make the system fit around you not try to fit around it."

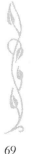

Be careful about these kind of maneuvers. It is possible to be caught and to lose benefits we might otherwise have qualified for or even to face legal sanctions. We really need good, often professional, advice when negotiating the social-service obstacle course.

For example, Medicaid provides good medical coverage, but to qualify a recipient must have almost no money. Social Security Disability Income is not "means-tested" like Medicaid is, but even it may be over the income Medicaid allows. We may need counseling to help make the hard decisions about what benefits to apply for. Inevitably, relying on such benefits will mean a more frugal way of life, but ways often exist to get stuff free or at a disability discount. For example, Oscar goes on extremely cheap rafting trips with a group called Healing Waters. A friend took him to Europe with his frequent-flier miles.

According to Oscar, when it comes to trying to get into programs, "You have to advocate for yourself socially and financially." Although others cannot understand our needs as well as we do, a friend or family member can still help advocate for us. We can all use someone who acts as advocate/bodyguard/secretary/attack dog when dealing with various bureaucracies and medical establishments. In many cities, AIDS groups have counselors who specialize in hooking people up with benefits, and such counseling services often are not restricted just to AIDS patients. Social workers in hospitals or service organizations can also help.

⌒ Help from Other Sources

In addition to help from family members, friends, and social-service agencies, other sources of support also exist. Pets provide a lot of comfort. Money can ease the burden; with it we can hire helpers, pay for treatments, and buy things to make life easier. One potential source of income is disability pay. Most of us don't want to go on disability, but it can be lifesaving. As Rob Mitchell's father told him, "You don't go on disability to die; you go on disability to heal." At the very least, such payments can keep us alive and can open opportunities for a decent quality of life.

Social Security Disability Insurance (SSDI) can be hard to get, but it can pay over twelve hundred dollars a month (the Social Security Administration will provide an estimate of the amount of your disability payments). Participation in SSDI can also confer Medicare coverage after a two-year waiting period. Thad Smith, a multiple-sclerosis peer counselor, stresses the importance of good documentation when trying to qualify for SSDI. "It is really important to have the support of your doctor and to see him or her regularly," he says. "You need documentation of things like fatigue or cognitive problems that prevent you from working." It may be helpful to get an attorney to represent you. There are attorneys who specialize in disability cases, and they advertise. Often, they only charge for their services if they are successful in obtaining benefits for the client. Check your local Yellow Pages.

Because SSDI payments rarely replace a full-time income, we will be much better off if we also have another form of disability insurance, either through our employer or privately. Some employers offer long-term-disability insurance benefits; Smith recommends we make such benefits a priority in our job search. But then we need to actually take advantage of the benefit, whatever our state of health. We never know when we will need it. "It's a safety net," Smith says. "I have seen coworkers who did not buy the insurance and then had cancer and were economically devastated."

We may be eligible for other benefits: low-cost meals, assistance with prescription drugs (from the government or the drug company), food stamps, help with phone or utility bills, various veterans' benefits. Scott Parkin of the National Council on Aging says, "There are close to a thousand benefits programs that people miss out on simply because they don't know about them." If you are a senior or on permanent disability, you can check out the website www.BenefitsCheckUp.org.

It doesn't hurt to ask government, charities, family, or friends for financial help. Perhaps we can also learn to value more highly the services we provide, if any, and charge more for our time when appropriate.

Online support is surprisingly useful. Chat rooms, newsgroups, websites, and mailing lists can be great sources of information and support (even though your online friends can't do the dishes for you). Beth remembers that the people she met online provided her with much information that has helped her cope with and heal from her condition.

We have inner support available to us through imagery and visualization (see Chapter 7). Finally, there is the totally reliable support of God.

However you may conceive of a higher power, such support is always available and often extremely valuable.

⌒ Plan for Help

My best advice is this: Don't let yourself get isolated in the first place. Get to know your neighbors, and befriend them at every opportunity. Improve communication with your family and friends to deepen those relationships. Don't be afraid to ask for help, and don't hesitate to give it, as long as you don't put your own needs on hold. Consider senior housing, if appropriate, and consider signing up in advance, because there is usually a long waiting list for the good housing. Remember, life is a team sport. Make sure you know where your teammates are.

Even with all the support in the world, we need reasons to do the work of getting and staying well. People have died despite the best medical care in the world, treatment that should have cured them but failed because they lacked the will to live. Most of the time the results aren't so spectacular or final, but the presence or absence of reasons to live often makes a huge difference in chronic conditions, as we will see in the next chapter.

TWENTY-FOUR
REASONS TO LIVE

*Ask yourself, what kind of life would make you glad to get up
in the morning, and glad to go to bed at night?*

Lawrence LeShan, *Cancer as a Turning Point*

SOMETIMES, A REASON TO LIVE costs $1.19 at K-Mart. That's
what researchers in a Connecticut nursing home found
when they divided the residents into two groups, roughly
similar in age and health status. Half the residents were given small
potted houseplants and told, more or less, "We're giving you this plant
to make your room look better. The staff will take care of it. Enjoy."
Members of the other group were allowed to choose their plant and were
told something like, "This is your plant. You take care of it, or not, as
you choose." This group was also encouraged to make other choices about
their living situations, for example, the arrangement of furniture in their
rooms.

Eighteen months later the death rate (among the humans) for the
"plant is your responsibility" group was less than half that of the "just look
at the pretty plant" group. Less than half as many of the group that was
given more responsibility had died! Now, caring for a houseplant is about

as minimal a purpose for living as you can get, yet doing so—as one part of being asked to choose certain aspects of their surroundings—apparently made a huge difference in this nursing home. The message is clear: People sicken or die each year because they can find no compelling reason to be well.

Without a reason to live, no one will seriously adopt self-care. Forget about it! It's too much work. Nor will our unconscious repair systems probably try very hard. So rather than waste a two hundred–page program for getting well, let's spend a chapter answering the question, "Why bother?" Health has potential value only because it can enable us to live richer, better, more fulfilling lives. If those lives aren't happening, what's the point? We might as well stay in bed.

Fortunately, reasons to live are not hard to find, as the nursing-home study shows. This chapter gives a lengthy but incomplete list of possibilities. All we need is one good one (although the more the better)—so nobody needs to try them all, no matter how "vital" I say some particular item is. And even if you feel quite in touch with your personal motivation for getting well, you might find some cool ideas here.

ᴇ What Am I Doing Here?

Most of us need some purpose in life, and it doesn't even have to be a very good one. At Mt. Zion Hospital in San Francisco, I took care of a woman with bone cancer who told me proudly that five years previously her doctor had given her six months to live. To his statement she replied, "I will go to your funeral, you bastard." Three years later she attended his burial and seemed quite pleased about it. Though she lived in constant pain, she was planning on burying a couple of more docs. It gave her something to look forward to.

Positive purposes usually work even better. My eighty-year-old friend Shirley has been bent over and hobbled with arthritis and scoliosis for forty years, yet she exercises, travels the world, keeps her own house, and remains active in a number of local, national, and international political causes. Her lifelong crusade for social justice as she sees it, a passion she shared with her late husband, seems to enable her to function at a capacity far beyond what any health-care professional would believe based on a physical examination.

Having an important cause gives us reason to live and get well, even if the cause is important only to us. Doing good at any level—for our country, city, community, neighborhood, or family—gives our heart a reason to pump, our joints a reason to heal, and our behinds a reason to get out of bed and move. And, purpose goes far beyond what we normally think of as doing good. It could be renovating a building, starting a business, helping raise grandchildren (or other people's children), writing a book, playing the conga drums, planting trees, keeping your sidewalk clean—a truly infinite variety of things. Involvement in the lives of our families, as caregiver, counselor, rooting section, or friend is a source of purpose that illness cannot take away. Even the role of recipient of your family's care is a chance to give them love and guidance.

The self-help section at the back of the book offers exercises for finding purpose as well as practices to help us clear away distractions, because a purpose can become a source of frustration if we don't act on it.

— *Work Necessary, Job Optional* —

Work should be a reliable source of purpose. Unfortunately, many of us labor in jobs we neither believe in or like, and this dissatisfaction can cost us dearly. Dr. Lawrence LeShan, in *Cancer as a Turning Point*, tells many powerful stories of people who recovered from apparently terminal cancer while moving into a job or way of life that better suited who they really were. He believes our bodies' defenses and recovery mechanisms work much better when we live and work in ways that express our deepest selves.

When we are out of work, as people with illness often are, it is helpful to find what the Presbyterians call a "place of usefulness" in the world. One of my more disabled MS acquaintances makes a partial living as a pet sitter. The animals and their owners love her because she gives them such undivided attention. She says, "It lets me know I'm still here."

Getting involved in helping others or doing some kind of volunteer work keeps some people healthy in situations where others drop under the weight of having no money and nothing to do. I love volunteering because you don't have to put up with any crabby bosses. You don't have to do things you know are wrong just because "it's always been done that way."

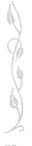

75

Being forced to help can become a burden, but help we choose to give tends to make us healthier and happier. There are hundreds of ways to help, some of which we can do from bed or over the phone. We can pick one, try it, and if it doesn't work, try something else.

⸺ *I'm Focused; You're Obsessed* ⸺

A caution about purpose: There is sometimes a thin line between focus and obsession. If I am so determined to finish my book that I cut back deeply on sleep, exercise, relaxation, and time with my family, the purpose may kill me instead of helping me to get well.

Mexican radio journalist Maria Victoria Llamas became deeply involved in a crusade to defend a woman named Claudia, charged with murdering a man who tried to rape her. As Maria Victoria wrote her book, *Claudia*, she began smoking and drinking coffee continuously through the day and late into the night to stay awake, and she began drinking alcohol to sleep. She didn't know she had the hepatitis C virus. It had never bothered her, but under the stress of her crusade for Claudia she ran her defenses down and almost died from the condition. Fortunately, she rested, stopped abusing her body, and with the help of friends, family, and several herbal medicines has recovered much, though not all, of her energy and health.

Purpose can also injure us if it is too open-ended and unachievable. "Saving the world," for example, is a purpose likely to do us more harm than good. However, fighting for a cause you care about—maybe saving a park, for example—can be achievable and can only help.

☞ More Meaningful Than We Know

Closely related to purpose is the idea of meaning, believing that our lives fit into a bigger story, a larger context. Because our society rarely speaks of meaning, we may not realize how important it is. Dr. Rachel Remen, author of *Kitchen Table Wisdom*, says, "We all live much more meaningful lives than we know." Being in touch with the meaning our lives have, for us and for those around us, can take us a long way toward getting well.

Seeing ourselves as part of something larger—family, community, ethnicity, cultural change, science, industry, or some other entity—puts our lives in a context that makes them more meaningful and tolerable. A worker may spend his or her day gluing together circuit boards he or she doesn't understand, but he or she may feel good knowing those boards are helping wire the world in a great telecommunications revolution. A parent may work twelve hours a day for low wages and barely know how to read, but he or she derives meaning from making sure his or her children will go to college and enjoy a better life. A disabled person may never make much money, but may be part of a movement that opens doors for others with disabilities or may act as a role model for others facing adversity.

— *Tell Me a Story* —

How do we get in touch with the sources of meaning in our lives? One valuable way is to tell our stories. Tell them verbally to others, put them on tape, or write them down in a journal. Get someone else, maybe of a younger generation, to help you make a video of yourself talking about your life. Think about where you came from, the times you've lived in, how they've influenced you, and you them. Remember the highs and lows, what you learned, whom you helped, and who helped you. You may find some real sources of strength, some reasons to value yourself, to care for yourself, to get well. Don't think, "Nobody's interested." Most people are nosy. But even if nobody else hears our story, it is good to tell it for our own benefit.

You can create a better life story if you remember more. Take time for memories, looking at pictures, going over old times with family and friends. A source of meaning for nearly all of us is the role of passing on culture and history to younger generations, and we also need memories to make sense of whatever is happening to us now. Memory is extremely fallible and fleeting, and its failings can leave us adrift and cut off in a sea of changing times. This is one good reason to take pictures and keep a journal—and also to pay more attention to life as it happens the first time. We'll have a better chance of remembering it.

⸺ *Faith and Spirit* ⸺

Religious belief is often a source of meaning for those who have it. Believing that God has a plan, that we are doing God's will, carrying out our karma, continuing the work of our ancestors, or moving towards a better existence in heaven or in another life can give us a sense of peace and certainty. Regular spiritual practice such as prayer or meditation may keep us centered and better able to focus on all the demands and opportunities of living.

Of course, we can't manufacture faith just because we know it's good for us, but it doesn't hurt to keep an open mind to the possibility. We all have spiritual beliefs, but many times we are unaware of them. Some of them can be quite destructive. Dr. O. Carl Simonton, author of *Getting Well Again*, notes that we may believe we will be forgotten after our deaths, that our lives have been meaningless, that we are unable to get well, or that we are doomed to burn in hell. Obviously, such beliefs make it difficult to stay healthy!

Dr. Simonton says that clarifying our basic beliefs becomes critical when we have health problems. Much pain and suffering that appears physical is actually spiritual, he says, related to fears about death and the value of our lives. Many of us are too embarrassed or uncomfortable to talk about these issues with our loved ones, but doing so will take a load off our hearts and minds. A good place to start might be with preparing advance directives (available at any hospital) for end-of-life care. That discussion tends to bring up a lot of spiritual issues, and having such a directive on file can save a lot of anguish later on.

As we have seen, it is possible to change our beliefs by conscious effort, and people who experience illness often develop faith as a result. Some people believe in God, some in Nature, others in science, art, humanity, love, or some kind of life force. We know that thinking and talking about the spiritual or metaphysical aspects of life is likely to bring us a sense of peace. If we are already part of a church or other religious affiliation, we might consider strengthening our involvement.

☞ What About Love?

Nobody has defined exactly what love is, but everyone wants more of it. Children and grandchildren, brothers and sisters, elders and other family members, friends, or pets can make us happy with their presence, their voice, their pictures on the refrigerator. Someone to love means someone to do things for, to look forward to, to think about. A good marriage or partnership makes a huge difference in longevity and health. (For men, that is. Married men, on average, live eight years longer than the unmarried kind. For women, the difference is so slim that no marriage at all is much better than a bad marriage.)

I had a client with heart failure who clearly seemed to be dying. She was in and out of the hospital every couple of weeks, her weight shot up and down like a Superball (a sign of fluid retention), and most days she was too weak to leave home. She went to church faithfully, though, and one day she met a man who fell in love with her. He proposed marriage, and she said, "Wait until I'm better." He said, "I don't want to wait; you might not get better." So they married, and she got somewhat better. Although still far from well, she stayed out of the hospital for months at a time and resumed a social life.

Dr. David Sobel writes that he has had many patients recover from high blood pressure, back pain, depression, and other conditions after falling in love. "Love, and its associated thoughts and feelings," he writes, "can dramatically reshape our minds and bodies, from organs to cells to molecules."

Easy to say, but presumably most of us would get more love if we knew how. How do we find love if we feel isolated, unworthy, unlovable, or just too busy? In interviews, literature, and my own life, I have found that love isn't something we find; it is an ability that we can develop and strengthen by practice. Be open to it, and it will find you.

First, and usually most difficult, we need to love ourselves (see Chapter 6). Then we can gradually start loving our families, friends, other people, and even animals, plants, or places more easily. We practice seeing the good in people and sympathizing with their struggles and problems, which are usually similar to ours. We can get better about recognizing and accepting the love of others. Love costs nothing to give and doesn't require a prescription to get. Best of all, no one and no change in our life situation—maybe not even death—can stop us from giving and receiving love.

This all sounds very spiritual and uplifting, but most of us want that one special person. Some ideas for improving a partnership, if you're in one, were given in Chapter 4. If your relationship is badly damaged, or if you seem unable as a couple to move beyond the stresses brought on by a chronic condition, you might consider working with a professional counselor or therapist.

If we don't have a partner, we often feel we will never find a good one, especially if we have illness or disability. We fear the pain of rejection, so we don't make ourselves available. With or without physical illness, it may take time to build our confidence to where we can envision finding someone. You will probably be amazed, however, to discover how many good potential partners are out there, even for those with health problems. Of course, we have to get involved in social situations to let them find us, but other people can often see the good qualities you can't see in yourself. One mixed blessing is that some people are looking for someone to take care of. Support groups or volunteer organizations are good places to meet good people. Ninety percent of finding someone is making oneself available.

Or, perhaps we remain attached to a former partner we have lost. Dealing with death or divorce takes time and support, and the process cannot be rushed. In the meantime, it is even more important to connect with family, friends, and other sources of love.

— *Love and Sex* —

Once, while working at Kaiser Permanente as a telephone advice nurse, I spoke with an elderly man who wanted a medication refill. He was taking a number of drugs for advanced cancer, chronic pain, and heart disease, but he didn't need those. He wanted more yohimbe, a West African herbal aphrodisiac.

Judith Sachs, in *The Healing Power of Sex*, wrote of a woman in the ICU who was lapsing in and out of a coma. Every time she woke up she asked to be given one of her birth control pills. When asked why, she said, "I plan to get out of here some day, and I want to be ready." Stories like these illustrate two points: the importance of sex and the excessive degree to which our society equates sex with erection and penetration. But anyone watching the stock of Pfizer, the company that makes Viagra, already knew these things.

Sex can be a wonderful reason to keep going when everything else seems bleak. It can be a way of connecting with someone we love, of giving our bodies attention, of relaxing, even of mild exercise. It's good for fatigue and excellent for pain relief. In addition, there really is no known illness that makes sex physically impossible, if we define sex not as intercourse but as physical contact for the purpose of sharing intimacy and pleasure. Stroking, kissing, looking, holding, talking sexy—these can all give the pleasure of sex without requiring intercourse. (And, of course, we now have a variety of medical interventions to make intercourse easier.) The body is full of sensitive places most of us never find because we don't look. By exploring the body for responsive areas, even quadriplegics can often enjoy good sex lives.

When we are sick or disabled, or consider ourselves disfigured, it is sometimes hard to imagine ourselves attractive even to a longtime lover, much less to someone new. But most people struggle with feeling unattractive despite the state of their health or the condition of their body. Your partner probably considers you much more attractive than you do.

Some couples benefit from counseling to help them deal with sexual relationship changes and other stresses caused by illness, and some counselors say the key to enjoying sex, with or without disability, is to relax. Let whatever happens happen. It's not a competition or a performance; it's a chance to connect with our bodies and our partners.

Of course, when we feel bad we may be less interested in physical contact. Depression, common with illness, may cause a lack of sexual interest, and that possibility should be explored if necessary. Sometimes, as with heart disease, there are concerns about safety. Don't feel pressured; not everyone needs sex, but everyone can benefit from contact. Foot rubs, neck rubs, holding hands, and hugging should feel like safe ways to start enjoying physical pleasure. Actually, except immediately after an acute heart attack, even vigorous sex is pretty safe if we take some simple precautions. It is believed that the number-one risk factor for cardiac death in men during sex, for example, is cheating on their wives. So you'll want to think twice before doing that!

☞ Keep Looking Ahead

Having something to look forward to keeps people alive. Death rates tend to drop in Jewish communities in the weeks leading up to the Passover feast and in Asian communities before the Moon Festival. After each holiday there is a compensatory rise. Until such time as we decide we no longer want to live, we may need to keep something in front of us to pull us along. A grandchild's wedding, the next election, whatever interests us in the future will tend to keep us going. As one goal nears, it's time to start looking for the next one.

☞ Pleasure Is Good for You

How many times have you heard that being healthy means giving up everything you like? All evidence shows the exact opposite. Give up the things you don't like, get more of the things you do, and find new ones that you like even more. There are hundreds of sources of pleasure, most of them readily available and safe, even if they seem to hide from us much of the time. Part of self-care is making sure we experience more of them!

What follows is a short list of potential sources of pleasure and energy. Nobody needs all of them; in fact, any one could be sufficient. Let's start with the five senses. In their landmark book, *Healthy Pleasures*, David Sobel and Robert Ornstein write, "Through pleasure, our senses guide us to experiences that enhance health. Sensory pleasure and positive mood is nature's way of letting us know that we are doing things that are contributing to our survival and our health." Consider some of the many sources of sensory pleasure:

Pay attention to the visual beauty around you—trees, birds, fish in an aquarium, flowers, children, good-looking adults, artwork, butterflies, the patterns on a leaf, attractive clothes, to name a few.

Listen to the sounds in the air—birdcalls, children's voices, the rush of wind or patter of rain, recorded music or nature sounds.

Notice all the delicious smells—coffee in the morning, bread baking, a fresh breeze. Lemon, garlic, lilacs, a light touch of perfume—pick your own medicine; thousands exist.

Enjoy the sensation of touch, especially affectionate touch; find a way to give and get more hugs. Feel different textures; take up a craft like pottery. Get an occasional massage from a professional or a loved one.

And don't forget your taste buds. We in richer countries now have access to foods from all over the world. Eating a variety of foods will deliver a full range of different and useful nutrients and new experiences, so try something new once in a while. A lot of foods we have been warned against actually aren't so bad. Chocolate has useful antioxidant effects, and even alcohol consumption, in moderation (one to two drinks per day), has been shown to reduce heart-disease risk by one-third.

~ *Appreciation* ~

Of course, none of these sensory pleasures do us any good if we don't notice them! We have to take time to taste the food, see the sights, and hear the sounds. Some people may need to limit salt intake but may really love potato chips. They can practice savoring one chip really slowly—getting the pleasure without eating dangerous quantities of salt. Some of us may need to learn selective attention, filtering out ugliness to focus on the good stuff. Unfortunately, many of us are better at doing the opposite, but we can learn.

~ *Fun Therapy* ~

The healing power of fun and laughter is well supported in theory, but many of us fail to get enough to test for ourselves. My mother-in-law, Rachel, says cartoonists and humorists are the unsung heroes of the world. This world is painful, but it's also funny, and since we can't avoid the former, we might as well enjoy the latter. Perhaps the healthiest form of laughter is laughing at ourselves.

One benefit of fun is that it requires us to stop taking ourselves too seriously. Try something we're not good at. If we feel too self-conscious to risk looking foolish, having a friend do it with us can give us confidence. People will admire us for trying. They may even be inspired to do something adventurous themselves. Games and puzzles are also good sources of pleasure, and they keep our minds active.

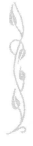

What can we do if we are too depressed or too self-conscious to laugh at ourselves, or even at others? Is there a video we can rent? A friend who knows how to make us laugh? Would some chocolate lift your spirits? If none of these bear any benefit, consider getting treatment for depression: therapy, exercise, or medication. Some of us have been raised to believe that fun is a waste of time because it's unproductive. Perhaps the people who taught us that fun is wasteful never had any, but we don't have to follow their unhealthy example.

⟶ *Treat Exercise As Pleasure* ⟵

I love to go to the gym, but I hate looking at the suffering faces of my fellow exercisers. If I had my way, people would treat exercise as an opportunity to take pleasure in their bodies and to have fun by playing games and trying new things. Adopting an attitude of "no pain, no gain" usually leads within a couple of months to "no exercise." My MS-related disabilities prevent me from playing basketball and soccer, which I loved. But when I'm in the pool doing water exercises, I can still enjoy movement, so that's what I do. I also get pleasure out of lifting weights and dancing—and when you see me dance, you'll get some fun out of it, too.

⟶ *The Incredible Power of Pets* ⟵

It's amazing what an animal around the house can do. Take my client, Joe Quinn, who lived with class IV congestive heart failure. He was short of breath even at complete rest, could not tolerate any exertion, and was not expected to live more than a few months. Joe was not the ideal patient. He smoked, drank, and ate whatever he wanted and damn the sodium content. He should have been dead. Even so, he had been in class IV for over a year when I met him, and he was still ticking along when I stopped working with him six months later.

What kept him going? His wonderful wife did everything she could for him, but she worked full-time outside the home and didn't give herself much credit for Joe's survival. In her opinion, credit was due the dog she had given Joe—against his will—and who stayed with him twenty-four hours a day. "He keeps Joe going," she said. "He watches him all the time, follows him everywhere. Joe loves him."

How much difference can an animal make in our lives? It's almost unbelievable. A 1995 study followed a group of about two hundred heart-attack survivors for two years. Dog owners had 80 percent less chance of suffering a new attack than subjects without dogs! (Cat owners showed no benefit.) According to cardiologist Shmuel Ravid this result is fairly typical.

Other studies have found similar, less dramatic pet benefits, including better control of blood pressure, fewer reports of minor health problems, and less feeling of social isolation. Pets give us someone to touch, someone to love, someone who needs us, an opening to talk to other people. Walking dogs provides exercise; watching fish or a bird gives us relaxation. Senior residences and nursing homes are increasingly allowing and encouraging pet ownership; they are convinced of the benefits, and their residents insist on them.

⟶ *Siesta Time* ⟵

Naps can make life more pleasurable, give us opportunities to relax, and be something to look forward to during the day. A large study in Greece found that men who took afternoon siestas were 30 to 50 percent less likely to have a heart attack than those who didn't. (The amount of nighttime sleep the subjects got didn't make a difference.) Obviously, some employers might need a little convincing on this score—refer them to the August 1987 issue of the *Lancet*, where the Greek study was reported—but if you can structure your life to allow naps, do it. You will probably find yourself more productive as well as healthier.

⟶ *Getting Our Hands Dirty* ⟵

Millions of people get pleasure and meaning from gardening. I'm not one of them, but it's easy to understand the joy of seeing things grow under our supervision. It's kind of like having children who never talk back. Gardening keeps us in touch with the miracle of life and also provides an excellent source of exercise. Even those with sharply limited mobility can garden with the help of widely available products for disabled gardeners. If we have no access to outside space, we can still enjoy window boxes and houseplants.

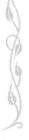

We must find a way to keep doing the things we love—gardening, cooking, or whatever our passion may be. We may have to modify the way we do it; we may have to buy some special equipment; we may need help. We may have to cut down on the amount of time we spend doing it, but we have to continue getting our hands dirty if that is what gives us enjoyment and fulfillment.

— *Go See Your Mother* —

Most people report feeling better after spending time in Nature, even in a little city park. Is it the quiet, the sweet smell of fresh air, the visual beauty, or what? One theory is that the natural world is timeless and therefore relaxing. Squirrels seem pretty busy, but at least you don't see them checking their wristwatches.

Sunshine is one of the benefits of getting outdoors. Sunlight helps our bodies create vitamin D, a shortage of which is now implicated by research in a number of illnesses. Sun exposure is known to lift depression, and it may confer other advantages. After all, our species has historically spent a lot more time outdoors than we do now, and our bodies may miss the sun more than we know. (Because of the risk of skin cancer, be sure to take precautions against overexposure.)

Some people believe that experiencing Nature helps us spiritually by reconnecting us with the Earth, where we came from. In Chinese medicine, living in accordance with Nature is the key to health, and isolation from it causes much of our disease. I believe it. The only time some of us see a tree is when we're driving past one while talking on a cell phone. I think the reason sex carries so much weight in this culture is because during sex is the only time many of us are in contact with a natural process or with our own bodies.

Far too many people never get out; their isolation from Nature is a form of oppression. In my hometown of San Francisco, thousands of poor kids have never seen the ocean though they live within a few miles of it. If we live too far from any green space or have severe mobility limitations, we may be able to get transportation help or learn to see the natural beauty in a backyard or small park.

Finding Some Comfort

As anyone with chronic pain can tell you, constant discomfort saps your energy like few other things. Severe pain is discussed in Chapter 7, but even when pain isn't severe, tension and minor annoyances (e.g., aches, itches, tightness) make us tired and interfere with our will to live and be well. Increasing our comfort level can provide health benefits, and doing so isn't always difficult.

First of all, do you have comfortable places to be: a decent bed with a proper mattress, chairs that fit your body? What about your car, if you have one? Do the seats feel good to sit in? And how about shoes and clothes? Are they too tight? How do you feel while wearing them? Sometimes it is helpful to change shoes every four to six hours, especially if you have circulation problems.

Comfort is partly a matter of attitude. Our minds can redirect themselves from parts that hurt to parts that feel good, or we can focus on an area of discomfort and relax it or compartmentalize it so it doesn't take over our whole consciousness. Over years of feeling miserable, some people become uncomfortable being comfortable. We have to believe it is okay for us to have some comfort in our lives.

Back to School

Self-care involves personal growth, that is, the development of new skills, attitudes, and parts of ourselves. The benefits of education, for example, are tremendous. A typical study on the subject, from Sweden, found that every type of illness and health problem, without exception, was more prevalent and more serious in people with fewer than twelve years of education than in those with more. Other studies have found that the more education you have, the healthier you are likelier to be, even when the studies control for financial status. Even people in their eighties who take classes or enroll in degree programs seem to do better—and to have reduced risk for Alzheimer's disease as well.

We don't need to go to a formal school to learn new things. We can take up new hobbies or explore new areas of knowledge. Learning makes us feel unstuck, that life still has new and positive things to offer. Most of the changes advocated in this book fall into the category of learning new skills, behaviors, and attitudes.

☙New Experiences

New experiences make life seem interesting and worth sticking around for. How about travel? Maybe we're not mobile enough or rich enough to take on the world, but aren't there places and people in our own city or country that we haven't seen? We may have to get help, of course. Millions of us unnecessarily limit our mobility because we don't want to go out in a wheelchair or use a cane or ask for a ride. Those of us who can't drive may not want to spend money on a cab, so we avoid going to places we would like to visit. Review Chapter 4 if you need to overcome a resistance to asking for help with transportation.

Try new foods, new games, new music, or new hobbies or rediscover things you used to love and then put aside. The world is full of interesting and weird activities, many of which offer events listed in the newspaper or on the World Wide Web (both available at public libraries). New people tend to have new ideas, so it's a good idea to meet some. Are we interested in community, cultural, or church events? Are there senior centers or other community centers accessible to us? When we are further along in age and disability, assisted-living or senior-housing facilities offer activities.

We get extra healing points for using our creative side. Musicians and visual artists tend to live long, healthy lives (if they don't starve). Getting well is a creative process in itself, but such efforts as painting, music, poetry, sewing, quilting, or auto detailing offer proven benefits in health, happiness, and longevity.

My mother's friend Barb was recently diagnosed with cancer at age seventy. She decided to try something new by becoming an actress. She enrolled in a full-time training program, which included several hours of vigorous dance each day. That will certainly keep her life from getting stale! (Though I hope she remembers to get enough rest.)

New skills come in all shapes and flavors. Some we may wish we didn't have, like learning to button clothes with one hand because the other doesn't work. Some are quite valuable and generalize to all areas of life, such as assertiveness, pacing ourselves, and other skills covered in this book. Some fall in between, like learning to cook tasty food without salt or learning efficient ways to keep house without getting exhausted. We can and should learn skills unrelated to our illness. Jacques, who lives up the street from me, was a star football player in his youth, until crippled by arthritis. He was bitter about it for thirty years, until he discovered table tennis. He took it up eagerly and represented the United States in the 2000 Paralympics in Australia.

Any reader who has slogged through all this wonderful stuff is probably convinced by now that life is worth living, at least in the abstract. Where it all falls apart for many of us is in disbelieving that we ourselves are worth living for. Raising the value we put on our lives comes partly from making them better and partly from raising our self-esteem. Valuing ourselves is part of taking responsibility, the topic of the next chapter.

GROWING UP
UNDER FIRE

*The notion that the focus of healing is lodged with
the physician is incorrect. It is lodged with the individual. . . .
If [a patient] looks completely outside himself for help,
he places an unreasonably large part of the burden on
the physician and may retard his own recovery.*

Dr. Norman Cousins, *The Healing Heart*

OFTEN THINK THE MOST CHALLENGING ASPECT of chronic conditions is how they force us to grow, to take responsibility for ourselves, when we'd rather let someone else—perhaps our mothers, lovers, or doctors—take care of us. But overcoming chronic illness is mostly a matter of self-care, which, by definition, we have to do for ourselves. Although we can't write our own medical orders or call every shot, we must take responsibility for our part. This means making sure we understand and approve the treatments we undergo. In particular, we should educate ourselves about our condition, monitor how our bodies are doing, and assert our right to make choices about our treatment. This chapter shows how to do these things, and it highlights the enormous importance of self-esteem in recovery.

In most conditions, for most people, the passive approach—going to a doctor, a series of doctors, or other healers and saying, "Fix me"—offers much less than a fifty-fifty chance of success. One large study of people with cancer found that only 22 percent of those who reacted passively were still alive after ten years, compared to 75 percent of those who reacted with a "fighting spirit." The difference in outcomes—though not necessarily in mortality—can be as great or greater in other conditions, particularly chronic ones.

The active approach doesn't suit everyone; a minority of us cope best by denial and avoidance. My father was one of those; not requesting so much as an explanation, he left all decisions regarding his cancer to his doctor. Dad always was a sweet guy—a salesman by trade, with lots of friends—but he wasn't much of a fighter. Although we urged him to get second opinions and try some alternative therapies, he would not question his oncologist. As a result, he received chemotherapy and radiation that other cancer specialists said had very little chance of success, treatments that caused complications and greatly increased his discomfort and kept him in the hospital for months without increasing his survival time.

Perhaps his way was right for him. His tumor was aggressive, he was a smoker, and his heredity seemed shot through with cancer-prone genes. Quite possibly nothing he could have done would have prolonged his survival, although he certainly could have saved himself—and his family—some unnecessary misery by foregoing useless treatment.

At about the same time my dad was ill, Katherine, a family friend, was also diagnosed with cancer. Her attitude was a bit different from his. She says, "I thought maybe the doctors didn't know anything. After all, it took them a year to diagnose me. They didn't figure out I had cancer until my leg broke. I just decided I was not going to listen to them; I was going to find out for myself what was wrong with me."

Katherine had surgery on her leg and took prescribed medical treatment, but she also followed diets and took supplements she'd learned about from reading and "through the grapevine." She "tried everything," moving to a home with fewer fumes and chemical emissions, visiting other doctors and healers. She even had herbal medications sent from Germany, until U.S. Customs stopped them. She says her "outrage" at interference

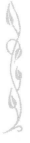

like that of the customs officials fueled her determination to get well by any means necessary. "It wasn't so much anger," she says. "I just believed the doctors were wrong in my case, and I was right."

Following her treatments, Katherine lived cancer free for twenty-five years; then she developed a different tumor, breast cancer. Again she had to fight, this time for conventional treatment—to get a mammogram and to start treatment when doctors said to wait. She feels she should have fought harder, but maybe she couldn't at her age, seventy-five. Even so, she is doing well.

Katherine had advantages, starting with an education at a women's college where "we all learned to speak up." She also had inherited some money, which enabled her to pursue alternative treatments. She believed in herself strongly enough to challenge a series of doctors and valued herself enough to make getting well the focus of her life. She had friends who supported her efforts even when her family didn't. Neither she nor anyone else can say whether her active approach made any difference. Still, the contrast in attitudes and results is striking.

☞ The Myth of the Exceptional Patient

Dr. Bernie Siegel, in *Love, Medicine and Miracles*, calls people like Katherine "exceptional patients." He writes, "Whatever they believe will help them get well that they can do, they will.... They are activists on their own behalf.... They seek second opinions, join support groups, and look into the alternatives." People who act in these ways tend to do better with any type of chronic condition, although how much better varies greatly from case to case.

"Exceptional patients" tend to be educated, self-confident, middle-class or above, with lots of support. However, there are exceptions to the typical "exceptional." Many of us don't have the strength, support, and opportunities Katherine enjoyed. The secret, though, is that we don't need to be "exceptional"—we only need to learn certain skills and attitudes, line up sufficient support, and commit to self-care. Sometimes the illness is too strong or our lives too hard for huge improvement, or perhaps lack of education, money, and social support may limit what we can do. Most important, though, are our sense of self-worth, our willingness to be

assertive, and the time we give to our bodies. If we learn and practice good habits in those areas, our results can be as "exceptional" as anyone else's.

⌒ More Control Than We Think

Medical science has developed the unfortunate view of treatment as a war between its medicine and our disease, with our bodies as ground zero. Instead of mobilizing our inner resources, this view tends to increase our stress with medically enforced passivity.

Norman Cousins, the prototypical "exceptional patient," refused to play a passive role in a losing battle. Editor of a national magazine, with many doctors among his personal friends, he overcame two chronic conditions: ankylosing spondylitis, an autoimmune disease that was supposed to kill him, and a major heart attack, which doctors said would require surgery and leave him disabled. To treat the spondylitis he relied mostly on laughter; after the heart attack he focused on exercise. He wrote books about each experience and inspired an informed public to demand more control over its medical management.

The latest science supports the idea of patient control. We used to hear that coronary artery blockage was irreversible and always required surgery. Now we know that self-care measures, attitude change, and social support can often open vessels or create new ones. We used to think that brain injury was forever; now we know that brains build new connections and even grow new cells. Biofeedback has shown that we have the power to increase our blood flow by voluntary thought and even to stop bleeding from wounds with the power of our minds. I have seen yogis stick barbecue skewers through their tongues without shedding a drop of blood; most of us would bleed for hours from a pinprick to the highly vascular tongue. I don't know *why* they do it, but it demonstrates that we have much more control over our bodies than we think.

Self-management—that is, educating patients to take more control of their conditions—has become the new watchword in chronic illness. We know that nursing-home patients who are allowed some choice over their environments live longer and that people who believe they control the course of their disease report fewer symptoms or complications. Some experts believe that many people find alternative medicine helpful because

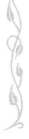

they choose it for themselves, rather than just following orders. More doctors now feel comfortable sharing knowledge and power with patients. Those who don't share need to be educated—or replaced with doctors who do.

It's hard for many of us to take leadership in our own health, partly because we hear from birth the message that we are inadequate to manage ourselves. We believe our bodies are fragile and our minds too uneducated to understand the mysteries of medicine. The television show "Sesame Street" for years had only one health skit, and it gave only one instruction: "Go see your doctor." (Thank you, letter B and number 3!) Drug companies and HMOs flood us with torrents of advertising proclaiming that they and only they can save our health. But they can't do as much as we can do for ourselves.

── *How Much Responsibility Can I Take?* ──

The first step in taking responsibility for our own recovery is self-monitoring: paying closer attention to our bodies. People can often prevent disabling back pain or headache if they recognize the symptoms early and adopt relaxation measures. Quick response in the form of medication or, sometimes, meditation can short-circuit angina in heart patients and severe wheezing in people with asthma. Some people with epilepsy can prevent a seizure by doing deep relaxation when they feel one coming on, or even stop seizures completely with self-hypnosis. Such effective self-management only works if we stay aware, stop what we're doing, and take care of ourselves when the need arises.

In many cases we need to monitor ourselves in more formal ways. Diabetics check their blood-sugar level; heart patients keep tabs on their weight; people with asthma monitor their peak flow (how much air can be pushed out in one breath); people with hypertension regularly check their blood pressure. Some conditions and medications require periodic blood tests, X rays, or examinations. With most other conditions, what's required is monitoring our symptoms to determine which activities, situations, foods, thoughts, places, or people make them better and which make them worse. Once we have this information, it's important that we embrace the former and avoid the latter.

Self-monitoring is critical to self-care. One of my clients had a brother who decided to treat his diabetes with Chinese herbal medicine. Unfortunately, he felt so good on these herbs that he stopped taking his insulin or checking his blood-sugar level. He kept saying he felt great—until the day before he died in a diabetic coma. His story doesn't mean the herbs weren't good for him; perhaps with insulin and close monitoring they would have helped. It does illustrate that we cannot afford carelessness about self-monitoring.

Dealing with Depression and Anxiety

Psychologist Darcy Cox points out that millions of people suffer from unrecognized depression and anxiety that can make their physical conditions worse. She says, "The biochemical changes caused by depression make it harder to take responsibility in chronic illness, and in some cases such changes make the disease progression worse." She suggests self-monitoring for the symptoms of depression: change in appetite or sleep pattern, loss of pleasure in things we used to like, increased social isolation, increased fatigue, suicidal thoughts, mental slowness, or frequent accidents. Although each of these symptoms can have other causes, if we experience more than one of them (particularly suicidal thoughts), we should report them to someone who can evaluate us for depression.

Anxiety and fear often accompany chronic conditions. Like depression, they hurt our quality of life and put stress on our bodies. Symptoms include cold sweats, feelings of panic, intestinal upsets, shaky hands, obsessive thoughts, and difficulty breathing. If we experience such symptoms frequently, we should get ourselves evaluated. Good medical, alternative, and self-care treatments are available for both depression and anxiety.

Learning Our Own Patterns

Self-monitoring is a process of self-discovery. I know now, after many years and several unnecessary attacks, that my MS gets worse if I let myself worry about someone else's problems, especially those of my grown children. No one else can stop me from stressing myself out over my kids, so I finally learned to help my kids without worrying about them.

We need to ask ourselves some questions: When do we get stressed, and how do we react to it? What triggers our asthma or our abdominal pain? When are we likely to skip our exercise or relaxation? What kinds of things tempt us to start drinking excessively? We have to get to know ourselves, and then we have to apply that knowledge.

Some people's chronic pain may flare up when they see too many people in a day; others may tend to skip their medicines when they get lonely. For some people, driving in traffic is like playing heart-attack roulette; tension, anger, and elevated blood pressure are part of their normal commute. If we recognize a pattern such as this, we have the responsibility to change either the situation or our response to it.

Arm Yourself with Knowledge

The first step in active self-management involves becoming informed about our condition. This education has gotten a lot easier in the Information Age. Now we can learn about health, disease, conventional and alternative treatments, medicines, side effects, and self-care options over the Internet, from books, and in popular magazines. If we don't have Internet access at home, most community libraries offer free access to the World Wide Web. Some medical schools or university libraries will allow laypeople to use their resources, including computers, medical journals, and textbooks (be sure to ask for needed help from the librarians). Make copies of relevant articles to show your doctors.

Most recognized health conditions have had dozens of books written about them. The best ones, like this one, often include the knowledge of medical professionals and of people actually living with the disease. New health journals, available online or by subscription, seem to start up every week. Disease-specific organizations, such as the American Heart Association or the American Cancer Society, distribute valuable information free of charge, although in many cases it tends to be weighted toward drugs and away from other options.

Other people who share our diagnosis can teach us. Unless we have a very rare problem or live in a very small community, we should be able to find someone who knows about our condition from firsthand experience. Support groups are information treasure chests; perhaps one exists

in your area. The Internet is full of online support groups, chat rooms, and bulletin boards for every conceivable health problem. Enlightened medical centers and doctors routinely connect patients with others who have done well with the same problems. Of course, not all centers are enlightened; we may have to push a little.

Medical professionals themselves are prime sources. In *Life with Chronic Illness*, Ariela Royer quotes a patient as saying, "I've gotten a world of information from every doctor I've ever been with, because I interrogate them. I am not bashful! I am not the kind that walks in, he takes my pulse and blood pressure, and I walk out. I learned a lot from all of them."

⁓ *Too Much Information?* ⁓

What do we do with a hundred sources full of words and concepts we haven't seen before? How do we evaluate what is right for us? In particular, how do we decide whether to pursue a particular conventional or alternative treatment? Stanford's Chronic Disease Self-Management Program lists a few questions to consider: How good is the information supporting a given treatment? Are studies available, and how convincing are they? Are the sources unbiased, or are they trying to sell us something? Would this treatment require giving up something important to our overall health (like the man who gave up his insulin or a diet that requires us to cut out carbohydrates or vegetables)? Does the treatment sound dangerous, overly expensive, or difficult to obtain? If the treatment is going to involve pain, disability, or expense, do we have people to support us through it? We have to weigh the potential drawbacks and benefits.

People without a scientific background may have difficulty evaluating the relative quality of research studies, which is one reason we cannot completely trust newspaper accounts of supposed medical breakthroughs. Most newspaper reporters aren't scientists. We can show such information to trusted health professionals or support groups or ask for help on the Internet. A friend of mine even corresponds by e-mail with the authors of studies he finds.

We can and should seek second opinions. A good doctor will not be upset about a patient's looking for more advice. Insurance companies may give us a little more trouble, but they can sometimes be convinced it's in their financial interest to make sure a proposed treatment option is the right one. We may have to fight them through our state regulatory agencies, or we may just have to pay for the second opinion out of our own pockets.

One tip: The source for a second opinion should usually be as different from the first source as possible. Doctors who share the same practice, the same facility, even the same town often share the same information, approaches, and beliefs about particular areas of medicine. It is helpful to seek another opinion from farther away.

⁀ Permission to Be Well

Before most of us will take any of these steps toward recovery, we have to convince ourselves we deserve it. Self-care takes a lot of time, and many of us don't feel free to spend time on ourselves. We believe we cannot rest when Uncle Phil needs us to take him shopping; we can't exercise when the kitchen needs cleaning.

Dr. Darcy Cox says, "In American culture people don't often take time for self-care. They can become very competitive, have a high drive to have power and money, or be wonderful caretakers of others, but we're not good at nurturing or taking care of ourselves."

My young friend Connie couldn't see a reason to take care of herself. She continued smoking despite horrific asthma that frequently landed her in the emergency room. Her older brother had died of asthma, but she didn't seem to care. Why not? Apparently she valued herself at flea-market rates. Her life didn't seem to be going anywhere. "I was mostly partying and hanging out," she remembers. Since she was on difficult terms with her mother and worked at a low-paying job without much chance of advancement, what was her motivation to change?

After a particularly bad attack, which forced her to breathe desperately through closed airways hour after hour until she nearly died—"I was ready to give up," she says. "I was tired of fighting for my life." She finally managed to quit smoking. Giving up cigarettes was hard, "like giving up a huge part of me." She succeeded in part because she established closer relations with her mom and also enrolled in community college, where she achieved success. Now she feels she's going places. "I feel much better about myself," she says. "My confidence has gone way up. I have more energy. When you feel healthier, you feel happier."

Many of us don't feel we are worth the time, energy, or especially the money it takes to get well. There are people who, when diagnosed with life-threatening illness, refuse treatment because they think their families could use the money better in other ways. Although this can sometimes be a rational decision—especially when expensive treatments only prolong suffering to no good end—we can also suffer from valuing ourselves too cheaply.

The pop-psychology term for this pattern is *low self-esteem*. If the next few pages run the risk of sounding like psychobabble, it's because low self-esteem can be crippling or fatal for one very simple, straightforward reason: The less time and attention we give ourselves, the worse our condition will probably become. Financial planners say, "Pay yourself first." They mean we should put savings away before we start paying other bills. When it comes to our health, we must put self-care first. We must schedule the time we need to attend to our health before spending it on other demands that can actually wait.

⟶ How Much Am I Worth? ⟵

Why do so many of us place such a low value on ourselves? Dr. Nathaniel Branden, one of the developers of self-esteem theory, has explained some of the causes. Much of the problem comes from childhood—from our parents, teachers, and classmates. If we get messages of inadequacy as kids, we may find them hard to outgrow. Sometimes we give these messages to ourselves. We judge ourselves by our mistakes and perceived failures; we compare ourselves to the models in the magazines or the corporate success stories sold by the media. Judging ourselves by material wealth also may produce feelings of worthlessness.

We may have endured experiences that cause us to see ourselves as unworthy. A history of physical, emotional, or sexual abuse can certainly do that, but a simple lack of attention from parents and others can also leave us feeling unimportant. A disability or illness that makes us look or act "different" can isolate us from others and make us feel worthless. We may have suffered discrimination based on ethnicity, sex, or some other characteristic and then taken on some of the negative attitudes we received from more dominant groups. All of these experiences can be overcome. Therapy may help, especially for survivors of abuse.

Health problems may lower our self-esteem further, particularly if we cannot earn much money. No matter how good we are as people, society tends to judge us, and we judge ourselves, based on our ability to pull economic weight. We may feel guilty for "making ourselves sick" or putting a burden on our families. This problem gets worse when we underestimate our abilities to recover. We, and our doctors, can boost our self-esteem and healing by stressing how much we are still capable of.

Is Feeling Good Selfish?

Whenever I teach self-care, someone always says they can't do it. "That would be selfish," they claim, if they have children or elderly parents or grandchildren or anyone else to take care of. "It's not productive," someone else may say. Relaxing or exercising (or doing anything for ourselves, such as having a little fun) doesn't get any work done or pay any bills. How can we justify the time and effort?

One way to resolve the conflict is to treat our bodies as if they were people who need help, just like others we care for. We can have enough compassion for our own bodies to let them rest or to give them the walk in the sunshine they desperately need, even if our minds are yelling, "Keep working!" Even in the economic terms of productivity, self-care is a good investment. If we enjoy more energy and better health, we will certainly be able to work better and to do more for others. We'll be in a better mood; our presence itself can be healing. Most of the great saints, healers, and spiritual teachers knew how to take care of themselves. Even Jesus got a foot massage; he rebuked Judas, who said the money spent on massage oil should have been spent on the poor.

Making martyrs of ourselves—ignoring our health to meet the world's endless demands—rarely does anyone any good. As religious counselor Wayne Muller says, our worn-down energy, cloaked resentment, and sense of hurry will outweigh most of our helpful acts. Of course, there are exceptions, when people may choose to sacrifice themselves for the common good. Some of us face enormous demands and decide to meet them consciously and with grace, even at the cost of our health and well-being. Most often, though, the choice is an unconscious one and is based on unhealthy beliefs about our self-worth and what it takes to be loved in this world.

⟶ *Forgiveness Begins at Home* ⟵

People who believe they are bad or worthless are unlikely to engage in self-care, and I believe their immune systems will also fail to repair damage or to fight enemies well. Dr. Branden says these negative feelings often stem from overgeneralizing and holding ourselves to unreasonable standards of perfection. Perhaps we consider ourselves lazy because we don't keep our kitchen as clean as our mother kept hers, when we actually work hard in other areas. If we harbor such attitudes, we tend not to give ourselves or others any slack for mistakes or shortcomings. We often talk about the value of acceptance and forgiveness, without making clear that it starts with us accepting ourselves. If we're doing something that violates our moral code, of course, we need to stop the damaging behavior, but many of us hate ourselves because we once said something mean to our dad or didn't finish college or don't look as attractive as we think we should.

Lots of us are living in private hells of guilt that we do not deserve but that make us sick anyway. Nursing professors Laura Meeks Festa and Inez Tuck relate the history of "Norm," whose brother died young in a car accident. Norm had blown up a paper bag and popped it; his father had turned around to yell at him and lost control of the car.

Norm blamed himself, perhaps with his parents' agreement. He developed alcoholism, which he kept under control for twenty years, long enough to provide for his family. A few years later, when the kids were grown and launched, Norm drank himself to death within one year. He never forgave himself for tragedies that were more others' responsibilities than his own.

Most of us carry around stories of pain we have caused, things we have done wrong, memories that weigh down our self-esteem. Usually the guilt is way out of proportion to the crimes. One of my clients developed severe back pain for which no specialist could find an effective treatment. The pain started when she put her mother in a nursing home; her guilt somehow seemed to localize in her back. The treatment involved realizing that she had had no choice; her mom needed more care than she could provide. When she accepted that fact, the pain subsided.

Dr. Branden says self-forgiveness comes from understanding the life situations that led to the guilt-causing behaviors. We always had reasons for our actions. If understanding why we did it doesn't help, we can try several steps: admitting we took the action; acknowledging whatever harm we have done, to the person who suffered the harm if possible; taking any possible actions to make amends or minimize the harm; and making a firm commitment to behave differently in the future.

We all tend to criticize ourselves over repeated mistakes and weaknesses. Society needs to recognize that nearly everyone is born with, or acquires at a young age, mental glitches, misperceptions, and minor disabilities that interfere with our lives. Everyone knows people who compulsively fall in love with the wrong type of person, consistently sabotage themselves in job situations, erroneously believe they are ugly or overweight—or some such pattern. We can see such areas of craziness in others, but our own often remain invisible to us. As we embrace self-care, we may come to recognize and correct some of our damaging patterns and learn to accept and compensate for other areas of weakness.

☜ *If You Were a Stock, I'd Buy Two Hundred Shares* ☜

How do we learn to value ourselves? In his book *How to Raise Your Self-Esteem,* Dr. Branden offers several ideas. For self-criticism such as "I'm lazy" or "I'm selfish," he asks us to identify times when we do not behave in these ways, when we show energy or generosity. By focusing on those times, we change the script to a more realistic one: We realize that we work or give some of the time and not others, like everyone else.

Dr. Branden's basic therapy involves sentence completion. He'll give a client a sentence stem such as, "I like myself most when _____" or "I like myself least when _____" or "One of the things I need to accept is _____." (He's got a million of them.) The client repeats the stem six to ten times and writes down whatever words pop up in his or her mind to finish the sentence. This is one way we can learn about our hidden thoughts—and then discard the ones that are unhealthy and out of sync with reality.

Other cognitive methods can help us develop healthy self-esteem. Affirmations are positive messages we can repeat to ourselves as needed, e.g., "I am getting better control of my asthma day by day" or "I am not perfect, but I am a good person and deserve to feel good." Make a list of all the positive adjectives you can honestly apply to yourself—use a thesaurus or dictionary if necessary or get a friend to help—and look at the list or say it out loud a couple of times a day. Review your successes and how you accomplished them. Try some of the exercises or read some of the books suggested in the Resources section of this book. Go see a therapist who specializes in self-esteem.

We don't exist in a vacuum; the attitudes of others influence our self-evaluation. We want to be around those who support us and point out our positives. We may have to look for and encourage such people, because some will react negatively. Don't expect a brass band and a party to celebrate our increased commitment to self-care, even if it is reflected in something as positive as quitting smoking. Our family and friends are used to us the way we have been, and our changing may make them uncomfortable for a while.

Stages of Acceptance

If we want to change something, we first have to accept it the way it is. When we have a chronic condition, accepting ourselves means accepting the condition, too. We keep hoping we'll wake up one morning and our problems will all be gone. We scan the papers for an announcement of a new drug or alternative treatment that cures whatever we have. Such announcements appear frequently, penned by gee-whiz science writers smitten with drug-company marketing releases, but they rarely pan out.

Eventually we have to accept some very hard things: This may never go away; it may get worse; I have lost or may lose some abilities I cherish; it is up to me to deal with this; perhaps, even, I may die from this. Some illnesses bring new losses that appear on no fixed schedule and have to be accepted all over again. Note that everyone, except those who die suddenly and young, must face these issues eventually. Even as a necessary part of growing older, accepting such things isn't easy.

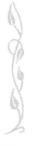

Margie Rietsma, one of Cheri Register's interview subjects in her book *The Chronic Illness Experience*, observed:

> When you lose [part of] your health with a chronic illness, you've lost part of you, just as if you'd lost a husband or wife. . . . People were pushing me so hard: accept, accept, accept. And they weren't giving me the time to mourn, to feel sorry for myself. . . . It's just like going through the death of someone. You have to go through all the steps, the whole process, before you can come back and do or be whatever you can without that thing you've lost.

Dr. George Solomon, who studied long-term AIDS survivors at Stanford, found that grief is indeed a critical step in the process of moving forward. Although long-term depression is unhealthy and unnecessarily painful, grief is good. It's okay, desirable in fact, to grieve even small losses; that's how we get to acceptance and then, hopefully, to action. There is no fixed timetable for getting to acceptance. Just know, even in the darkest hours, that it will come, and that you will get moving again.

⟾ *Accept and Fight Back* ⟾

Acceptance has gotten a bad name in some circles because people equate it with giving up. People think acceptance means dying in peace.

Dying in peace is good; everyone should die in peace. But living in peace is ten times more wonderful; it makes our presence in the world a blessing. I believe we can accept reality and still fight to get well—if we value ourselves sufficiently.

Acceptance poses special challenges when our condition is socially unacceptable, when our diagnosis is a source of shame or leads to isolation or discrimination. This used to be the case, and sometimes still is, with cancer and AIDS; it is now especially true of psychiatric conditions. Some of these have awful names—such as borderline personality disorder or schizophrenia—that imply personal failure, inadequacy, or danger.

Hard as it is, accepting the situation and taking responsibility is the best chance those of us with psychiatric conditions have. Some brave souls with severe problems like manic depression or borderline personality dis-

order have started their own magazines, websites, and online or in-person support groups. These groups do great things. Psychiatric disorders are ongoing health problems similar in most ways to MS, arthritis, and heart disease. They respond to treatment—if we take some control over our recovery.

Healing in Hell

Some people manage to embrace self-care in truly terrible situations. One of those people is my friend Marlon, who has spent the last seventeen years in California state prisons. In 1984, he killed a man in a fistfight over money and wound up with a second-degree-murder conviction and a sentence of fifteen years to life.

I met Marlon while he was playing in a band in 1983. He was talented and intelligent, but highly undisciplined. He never made much money with his music; he was too busy enjoying himself. In prison, though, there is little to enjoy. Inmates live in constant fear of guards and other prisoners and are lucky if they have one friend they can talk to. Even then it is dangerous to share feelings or show any vulnerability. Prisons are not for healing.

Five years ago Marlon tested positive for HIV, the virus that causes AIDS. The change in Marlon since he learned the results of that blood test seems remarkable. He immediately set out to "learn any- and everything I could about it. Not just the virus, but the medication, the side effects, everything. So I immediately started training myself in all aspects of it, which was phase one."

He continues, "I started applying those things that would keep me away from the medications," noting that the prison health service is often an unreliable place to obtain sensitive AIDS drugs, which must be taken at regular times every day. "Things such as eating better, exercising, trying not to stress, getting a good night's rest, taking vitamins. Everything except the stress part has been working for me, as the environment is extremely stressful! Even with the stress, I've been doing great in my fight against the HIV."

The sense of self-mastery and accomplishment I hear in Marlon's letters astounds me. This is the first time he has taken full responsibility for himself—had he done so earlier, he might not be where he is—and he has changed his attitude to life dramatically, even achieving a measure

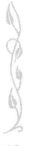

of serenity since his diagnosis. It helps that he has few symptoms, but he also has no support, professional or personal, in dealing with the pain of his life or the demands of his condition.

Marlon believes his exercise program, improved diet, and better attitude will enable him to fend off AIDS indefinitely without medication. This would be unusual, but his HIV virus level has been going down, and his T-cell counts (T-cells are the white blood cells attacked by HIV) have been going up, so who knows? He still has the option to start medication if he needs it.

He has come a long way in terms of maturity, he feels a lot better about himself, and he tries to help other inmates deal with HIV and prison life. These are not small things; they are terrific accomplishments in the poisonous atmosphere of the prison system. If my friend Marlon can heal himself to this degree in his barren wasteland, then no one should give up hope of healing, ever.

☞ Never Too Early or Too Late

When Juan Valenzuela got cancer at age eight, he had no one to fight for him. His parents spoke no English and were paid little respect by the hospital staff in New York. Juan says he learned to stand up for himself, became the "terror of the pediatric staff," went through two years of treatment, and wound up starting a support group for children with cancer—all when he was only twelve. Now he has hepatitis C, contracted from transfusions he received during his fight with cancer. He approaches hepatitis in the same active way.

A neighbor of ours, Sam, was born with developmental disabilities. Instead of trying to make his life as normal as possible, his parents kept him inside and did everything for him, so he learned little and made no friends. Recently his mother died, and his aging father became too disabled to care for him. At sixty-two, unable to tie his shoes or speak in sentences, Sam was sent to a residence program for the developmentally disabled. In less than two years he has learned a host of new skills, and he now has a girlfriend and a real life.

These two cases are not atypical. Forced by increasing disability to move to assisted-living centers, people whose lives have been closing in for decades suddenly start to flourish. Children and adolescents regularly survive challenges and suffering that seem insurmountable, and they seem to come out stronger for the experience. Stories like theirs confirm that nearly everyone is worthy and capable of living well, even with disabilities and chronic problems. The next chapter makes the case that our bodies are also worthy of love and respect, and that developing a closer relationship with them will improve our lives and health.

7

YOUR BODY—
LOVE IT OR LEAVE IT

*When I was lying in bed, just wanting to die, I "saw"
this little girl, who was kind of in my diaphragm, and she was
all ragged, and her hair was a mess, and she told me, "You've
starved me for years, for years." When I saw that, my whole idea
of my body having betrayed me completely changed.
And I saw that it was I who had betrayed it, and I said,
"I will never, ever not take care of you again."*

Arthritis conqueror Darlene Cohen

MANY PEOPLE'S BODIES probably feel like the girl in Cohen's vision, ignored and deprived. In his book *My Year Off*, stroke survivor Robert McCrum writes, "As adults, we forget that we live in our bodies." How is that possible? It sounds ridiculous. "Let me see, I've been so busy," I imagine someone saying. "Did I remember to bring my body today?"

But McCrum is right, and he doesn't go far enough. We don't just forget our bodies; we abuse them. And we don't just live in them; our bodies are a very large part of who we are. They are our major source of pleasure, and they are our interface with the rest of the world. The energy of life flows through them as we breathe, eat, and absorb the warmth of the sun. They enable us to reproduce and keep the circle of life going.

Yet many of us treat our bodies as we would a used car—and not a certified late-model Mercedes Benz, either, more like some two-hundred-dollar junker from the back of the lot, not worth even a regular oil change. We expect them to work and play and absorb whatever we throw at them without complaining, and when they break down, we think a mechanic with a medical degree will fix them. We treat them, in fact, the way society treats us: as agents of production, valuable only for what we can do, not for who we are.

Bodies are not machines. They are intelligent, living systems, and though they sometimes suffer, make mistakes, and need help, they know when and what we should eat, when we need to move and when to rest, and more. Boasting billions of connections with our brain, they are marvelously capable of memory, communication, emotion, and self-repair. Yet religion, science, and culture treat the body as an inanimate object or worse. Our major religions regard soul and mind as divine, but body as a source of temptation, even as something evil or disgusting. Science regards bodies as passive objects to be investigated, while business recognizes them as a source of potential profit.

Society prefers to ignore the old wisdom and new research showing that there is no place where "mind" stops and "body" starts. The body is shot through with mind; the nervous system transmits messages to and from every tissue in the body, maybe every cell. The entire body is alive, alert, and hopefully working for maximum health and fulfillment. This chapter celebrates the body's intelligence and demonstrates that loving, respecting, and listening to our bodies will help us get well.

Lost Connections

As children we have strong connections with our bodies, but we later learn to live entirely in our heads. When we renew our body connections and start treating the body as a friend, we also reconnect with a force that can help us live richer, healthier lives.

Cautionary note: While statements in other chapters, strange or not, are backed by solid scientific research, this chapter is more radical. Some of its content is based on preliminary research, some on anecdotes; some is speculative, spiritual, even poetic. If you are the skeptical type, you may want to translate part of what I say here into more conventional language—or just skip ahead. When I write about the body knowing, remembering, thinking, feeling, and communicating, you can translate that to mean that parts of our minds—parts with which we may be out of touch—are doing those things. We will even discuss how we can contact those parts.

Since all parts of the body communicate with each other through an array of chemical signals, and since the brain is part of the body, it doesn't make much sense even to talk about mind and body as separate entities. The phrase "mind/body connection" doesn't begin to do justice to what is essentially one unified "body/mind" or "mind/body." But it doesn't matter so much what terms we use. The point is this: Our bodies (or unheard parts of our minds) know what we need to do to live and get well. Parts of them may be in pain or malfunctioning or fighting some disease, but we need them, and they need us to give them support. The rest of this section gives examples of the body's apparent intelligence.

⌐ *The Body Remembers* ⌐

People who work with bodies, such as massage therapists, frequently have the experience of pressing on a tight muscle or other body part and eliciting a vivid memory from the client. Especially when working with deep pressure on ligaments and tendons, it is common for a client to get sudden memories of some long-ago event loaded with emotion. Don Johnson, who practices "structural integration," reports that some clients, during deep massage, have remembered experiences such as falling into a lake or being hit with a ruler. It seems the body may act together with the brain to keep buried memories alive.

If nothing else, the body remembers how to do things. As the saying goes, you never forget how to ride a bicycle. Some stroke victims lose the ability to describe their family house or to tell you how to move around in it, even if their ability to speak is okay. They don't consciously remember what their homes look like. But their bodies—or, if you prefer, unconscious parts of their minds—will still take them where they want to go. Some organ-transplant recipients tell of acquiring new memories along

with their new hearts or kidneys. While these reports are controversial, it is hard to explain all of them away.

— *Where Does Emotion Come From?* —

Most of us have had the experience of heartache, that heavy feeling around the chest that arises when dealing with loss. Until the late twentieth century, it was widely accepted that emotions originate in the body. We use the phrase "gut feeling" to describe the experience of "knowing" something based on our emotional response. Chinese medicine assigns a different organ to each emotion: The liver relates to anger, the kidney to fear, the heart to joy, the lungs to grief. In recent times, Western science has attributed all emotion to processes in the brain, but this idea is wrong.

Dr. Candace Pert, one of the founders of mind/body medicine (or psychoneuroimmunology), discovered some of the chemicals, called neuropeptides, associated with emotion. She and her associates identified emotions as biochemical reactions, each emotion with its own characteristic molecules. She also found that cells in all parts of the body contained receptors for these molecules. In other words, every part of the body feels our emotional state. This explains the white blood cells of the bereaved Australians from Chapter 1 that refused to fight their natural enemies (see page 6). Those cells were depressed.

Dr. Brent Atkinson, a psychologist, has studied the physical manifestations of emotion. He writes, "The body is the voice of the emotions, eloquently communicating critical information about our current emotional state. Tightened muscles and a sick sensation in the gut, for example, typically accompany fear, while rage is characterized by an upsurge in aggressive energy and increased body temperature."

— *The Body Wakes Us Up* —

Our bodies know when we're planning to do something stupid. Psychologist Harriet Lerner wrote about planning to marry a man about whom she had severe doubts. A few days before the wedding she awoke completely paralyzed, unable to move at all, a state that lasted quite some time. "I knew then," she writes, "I could never marry that man."

Diseases often play the role of wake-up caller. Robert McCrum writes of finding the meaning in his stroke:

> Since the doctors had failed to find a reliable explanation for my stroke, I came to the conclusion that it happened as the outcome of a profound internal dissatisfaction with my way of life.... The truth is that in my old life as a fit person I had become a monster of irresponsibility. For years I had lived for my freedom.... I reveled in ways of escape.... In hospital, I'd come to recognize that I'd been ambushed by the adventure I'd been looking for, and was traveling into a new and strange interior: my heart.

In my own case, I feel certain that MS is at least in part a response to my predisease lifestyle of running madly around, trying to do twelve things at once, screwing most of them up. My immune system forced me to slow down and focus, allowing me a much more satisfying life. One of my friends had given up working as a preschool teacher, which he loved, to pursue a more lucrative business, which took up all his time but gave him much less satisfaction. After his heart attack he returned to teaching preschool (and began exercising and changed his diet), and he feels his life is better than it has been in decades.

Bodies know our financial status. Research has shown repeatedly that compensated injuries—injuries we receive payment for—heal much more slowly. We don't just report more pain; our bodies actually take longer to recover. And when legal action is involved, injuries rarely resolve until the case is finished, if then. This usually does not mean we are faking, but rather that the body/mind can add and subtract the costs and benefits of healing.

The Incredible Immune System

Although it can get sick and cause illnesses of its own, the immune system acts in undeniably intelligent ways, more sophisticated than any human police force. It includes cells that "arrest" invaders and swim around searching for other cells that do the actual destroying. Still other cells generate chemical substances called antibodies to help fight cellular enemies. Others start inflammatory responses to control infection, while still others tell the system to back off when the danger is over. Most of these cells, and the organs that produce them, are in constant communication with the brain, and they are sensitive to emotional states and stress.

White blood cells in the immune system manufacture chemicals that affect our brains by, for example, making us more or less sleepy, which may be why colds make us want to rest. The immune cells also make a number of chemicals used to communicate with each other and the rest of the body. Immune memory goes on for decades. After a vaccination or during infectious illness, we produce large numbers of lymphocytes programmed to destroy the invading agent. As years go by and no new invasion occurs, the immune system will produce fewer and fewer of these cells, but it will nearly always keep a few around just in case. If the disease germ comes along, the remaining coded cells will identify the invader and reproduce rapidly to meet the challenge.

⟶ *The Body Goes Food Shopping* ⟵

Our bodies know what kinds of foods we need. If we give young children a wide assortment of food options and let them pick their own, they may pick some very weird menus. Over time, though, they will usually choose a completely balanced diet. Adult bodies also have this ability, if we pay attention. Geneen Roth, author of *When Food Is Love*, teaches seminars on living without dieting. She says healthy eating involves only two steps: "Eat whatever your body wants, and stop when you are full." We may have to modify this slightly if we have diabetes, and we must tune in to our bodies well enough to hear them instead of listening to our emotional needs or to the fast-food ads on television. Still, no one knows better than our own bodies what we should eat.

⟋ What Does Illness Want?

If the body has memory and emotion (or if the body at least holds them for the brain) and if it tries to communicate them, perhaps we should listen. Our bodies care about us and want us to experience pleasure and happiness. That's because when we are relaxed, comfortable, and happy, our bodies will be getting the oxygen, food, and rest they need.

When we are endangered or something is making us miserable, our bodies try to get our attention, but they are at a big disadvantage. They don't speak in words, so they have to communicate with emotions and symptoms, or sometimes in cravings or dreams, which we might misinterpret, ignore, or try to suppress. When we have health problems, whether headaches, heart attacks, or anything else, it is valuable to ask ourselves, "What does my body need? What does this symptom or illness want from me?"

The answers vary widely, but certain themes keep recurring. One common message, described in Chapter 2, is "Slow down." Another, discussed in Chapter 6, is "Love yourself more." A message that nearly all bodies try to send is "Pay attention to me!" Other common ones include "Get help" or "Let go [of some harmful feeling]." Sometimes the message is more complicated. But how do we talk to a headache? How do we listen to diabetes or cancer? We have to start by paying attention to symptoms.

Often when we have pain or other unpleasant symptoms, we go to a doctor or other healer and say, "Make them go away." Dr. Martin Rossman, author of *Guided Imagery for Self-Healing*, calls this behavior shortsighted. He asks, "If a warning light came on in your car, would you go to a mechanic and say, 'Rip out the light?' Or tape over it so you could go about your business? Probably not. You'd want to know what was going on under the hood. Then why go to a doctor looking only for relief of symptoms?"

A particular infection may be cured with antibiotics, a pain relieved with narcotics, or mood elevated with antidepressants, but if the underlying message isn't addressed, the problems will return in greater force.

Symptoms can communicate our deepest feelings, writes Debbie Shapiro in *Your Body Speaks Your Mind*. Sometimes the body does this poetically, she says. For example, pain in our upper back and knees, the weight-bearing areas, can indicate that we are carrying too many burdens with too little help. Frequent chest infections or pain may indicate that we need to "get something off our chests," such as grief or other unexpressed emotion. "Symptoms are not the enemy," says Dr. Rossman. Just as pleasure serves to draw us toward experiences that are good for us, symptoms exist to move us away from activities, feelings, and situations that harm us.

☞Imagery: Language of the Body

To hear what our bodies are trying to say, we often need to be quiet. Time spent relaxing or meditating or listening to quiet music may allow us to hear thoughts that we normally drown out. The body also communicates in dreams. Marc Ian Barasch writes in *Healing Dreams* of the long series of nightmares he had about terrible things happening to his neck—bullets in the throat, a pot of burning coals suspended from his chin by torturers—very scary images. He went to several doctors to report this, but, skeptical as most of us would be, they performed only superficial neck exams and found nothing. The dreams continued, and he kept going back to the doctors. He was finally diagnosed with a thyroid cancer that would have killed him had it gone untreated much longer.

How do we interpret nonverbal messages such as dreams or recurrent physical or emotional symptoms? Growing numbers of doctors, nurses, therapists, and laypeople are finding imagery an excellent way to hear the body's messages. Remember that only part of the brain (usually located in the left cerebral cortex) is verbal. This part thinks of itself as "I" and calls itself by our name, and we believe it, while the larger nonverbal parts of the brain may go unheard. Much of our inner wisdom, knowledge, and memory are unavailable to our verbal minds, but we can often gain access to this information through imagery.

Sometimes, as in Darlene Cohen's story at the opening of the chapter, these images come spontaneously. If we don't have spontaneous experiences like Cohen's or powerful dreams like Barasch's, interactive guided imagery (IGI) can give voice to the hidden parts of our minds and bodies. By using the imaginative and sensory parts of our brains, we reduce the control of the "I" part and allow other parts to be heard. During IGI, a tape or a human guide helps us to relax and get in touch with images for whatever problem we want to explore. People who feel uncomfortable closing their eyes and imagining can draw pictures of their symptoms or problems. Once we get our imagination going, we can hold "conversations" with these images in order to hear their messages.

☞ *Lifesaving Messages* ☞

At times the lesson is delivered with great elegance and creativity. Dr. Rossman saw one patient, a hard-driving fifty-something executive with diabetes, referred by his doctor because he refused to exercise or watch his diet. Rossman asked the patient to create an image in his mind for his diabetes. What came up for the man was a big, black ball and chain.

With Dr. Rossman's encouragement, the executive conversed with this image, telling it how much he hated it, that it was tying him down, and he couldn't accept it. When he listened for the image's response, he heard that it was crying. It didn't want to ruin his life, but it was tired. It couldn't go on, and it needed help. With more prodding from Rossman, the man asked what kind of help the image needed. When he looked again at the image, the ball had turned into a dog, and the chain into a leash! The dog needed to go for a walk, and it needed nutritious dog food, more water to drink, and a nap once a day.

"Could you do that for the dog?" asked Rossman. The man agreed and left with a commitment to give the dog what it needed in exchange for feeling better himself. During follow-up, the client indicated that while he still felt limited by his diabetes, he hadn't felt so good in fifteen years, and he planned to continue giving his imaginary dog real walks!

☞ *Straight from the Heart* ☞

Other people receive profound messages about their lives. One man, an Episcopal priest, had such badly blocked coronary arteries that he could not stand in a cafeteria line holding an empty tray without severe chest pain. He had already undergone two bypass surgeries; he was taking several medicines, following an extremely low-fat diet, and doing cardiac rehabilitation exercises, all without relief from the pain or change in his blocked arteries.

The priest attended a retreat and participated in a group experience with Dr. Rossman, who asked participants to have a conversation with their hearts. The priest's first response was, "No way," but eventually he agreed to consider a slightly revised version of the request: "If I were going to talk to my heart, what would I say?"

He wrote, "I found myself saying to my heart, 'I'm sorry.' In an instant, I was in tears and carried on a conversation with my heart, apologizing for having carried so much pain, sorrow, guilt, and grief in my heart. At the end of the dialogue, my heart told me, 'It's okay—I am going to keep beating.' And since that moment I have had no chest pain of any sort."

He reports that his cholesterol and blood pressure are down, his arteries show less blockage, and he wrote to me recently that his doctor hopes to have him off most of his medicines within a year. Yes, this stuff happens, though I have absolutely no idea what the physiological or psychological mechanisms are. Such stories show how healing may involve much more than diet, exercise, or medication. It often requires love and compassion, particularly for our bodies.

Who's Driving the Car?

Does it sound crazy to think of having multiple "parts" inside you, of having a conversation with your kidney, your fear, or some other part? Consider my mother's fairly common experience. She was driving on the freeway, deep in thought about problems at work. When she came back to reality, she had missed her exit and was ten miles down the road. Dinner was late that night! But the question Mom kept asking herself and anyone who would listen was, "While I was lost in thought, who was driving the car?"

We all know the feeling of being "of two minds" about something. For instance, most of us have a part that wants to be financially secure, another that wants to do good, and another that just wants to relax. Most of us have gotten ourselves into some kind of trouble with actions or words and have wondered, "What was I thinking? Where did that come from?" We really aren't sure, perhaps because some subconscious part was doing the thinking at that moment. Hypnotized subjects can be told they are temporarily deaf, and they will not react at all to a loud noise next to their ear. When they wake up, though, they can recall the sound, indicating that at least part of them did not buy the deafness suggestion.

Anesthetized surgery patients have demonstrated recall of things said in the operating room. Those told that they would wake up hungry and with relaxed muscles tend to have faster return of bowel function and less

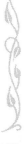

pain. (Audiotapes of similar suggestions to listen to before and during surgery are available, or we can make our own.)

When someone comes to me for help to stop smoking, I usually have the client create images for both parts of themselves: the part that wants to smoke and the part that wants to quit. The two parts can then talk it out; the client learns a lot more about what is going on and usually leaves after a few sessions with a good plan to meet both parts' needs without smoking.

Italian psychiatrist Roberto Assagioli writes that we all have various subpersonalities, and our task is getting them to work together. Whether we accept that concept or not, we are all much more complicated and multifaceted than we realize. It is better to get in touch with various parts of ourselves, because aspects we ignore or suppress will still fight to get their needs met, sometimes by making us miserable, self-sabotaging, or even causing illness.

⌒ Tired + Hungry = Mean and Nasty

Every parent and preschool teacher has had the experience of trying to quiet children who fuss, cry, or act out uncontrollably. We use all our creativity to distract them and our love to soothe them, and it works for about ten seconds. Then they start up again. What does that mean? It means they are hungry and/or tired. Until they get food or a nap, they will stay miserable and make us pretty crazy, too.

We can see this dynamic so easily in children, yet we tend to forget it when it comes to adults. When we find ourselves making a lot of mistakes, we are probably tired or taxed with too many demands. When we get grouchy and snap at people, even those we love, maybe we are hungry or need a nap. (And, when someone yells at us maybe they just need a banana or a back rub—not an argument or a major life change.)

Drug-rehabilitation counselors have learned that people do destructive things when they need sleep or food. They use the acronym **H.A.L.T.**, a reminder when patients feel in danger of using drugs, that they should instead stop and ask themselves if they're really **h**ungry, **a**ngry, **l**onely, or **t**ired. How much more empowering this is than the view we usually believe: that our reactions flow from some source in the outer world. We think

"outside sources" are making us angry when what we really need is to rest or eat. We push the body aside to meet the latest, often self-imposed deadline, and by so doing we come to see the world as a much more unpleasant place than it is.

Pain: The Mind/Body's Tightest Link

Chronic pain is the industrial world's most common and most expensive disorder. Low back pain alone generates twenty million doctor visits a year, and that doesn't include appointments with chiropractors, acupuncturists, and others whose livelihoods depend on patients in pain. Yet there is no medical explanation for the growing prevalence of severe pain. There has not been an increase in trauma, and there is no reason to think modern people are weaker or wimpier than former generations. What causes all this pain, and what can we do about it?

If we hit our finger with a hammer, pressure on nerve endings, swelling, and inflammation will cause sensations of pain that may last a few minutes, then stay around at lower levels for a few days. This is an example of acute pain, which reflects disruption of a body part. It normally goes away quickly. Even a fractured femur, the largest bone in the body, usually stops hurting in about six weeks, with treatment.

Most long-term pain, such as chronic back pain, stomachache, joint pain, or headache, does not indicate any ongoing damage to tissues at all. But in no way does this mean the pain is "all in our head"! Many experts believe we experience pain through a pain-recognition system, which links all parts of our bodies and minds and warns us of danger, as pain was meant to do. The pain and danger may be physical or psychic, or a combination. Our pain-recognition system can't tell the difference; in fact, physical pain often occurs together with depression and/or anxiety, psychic forms of pain. Pain and fatigue are where mind and body are most tightly bound up.

Pain specialist David Bresler says, "It is nonsensical to wonder if a patient has 'real' versus 'unreal' (imaginary) pain, 'organic' versus 'psychologic' pain, or 'legitimate' versus 'hysterical' pain. Pain is an intensely personal experience, and even if no physical explanation for it can be found, all pain is real."

When we have pain in excess of what any tissue damage should cause, we may have a disorder of the pain system, a warning of some other process that needs attending, or both. We can and must deal with the whole situation to get relief. Pain medication can be valuable, but Dr. Bresler points out that narcotic medications compete for nerve endings with the body's own painkillers, the endorphins, which are more effective. (Antidepressant drugs may work better; they don't compete with endorphins like narcotics do.) Bresler believes a treatment goal should be a reduction of pain meds and an increase in our internal pain-control mechanisms. Most important, he says, is to address the physical, emotional, and spiritual causes of the pain.

Imagery can help us control the pain and hear its message. We can imagine we have a volume control for the pain, which we can turn down to a tolerable level. We can imagine a place without pain or a time before the pain came or after it leaves. We can dialogue with the pain, asking it what it needs and what we can do to get some relief. It may even help to pay more attention to the pain, describing the feelings in detail, drawing pictures of it, becoming aware of other feelings that go along with it. The worst thing is often to fight against it, because doing so involves tensing all the muscles around the pain, which makes it worse.

We can also use body awareness to reduce the share of our attention the pain is grabbing, by learning to feel other things at the same time. We can note areas that are relaxed, soft, hard, tense, hot, or any sensation other than the pain. We can explore the pain: Is it sharp, dull, hot? Awareness Through Movement, also known as Feldenkrais, is used in growing numbers of pain programs. Feldenkrais teachers help people to make small movements, remaining aware of the feelings created and finding ways to move that don't hurt. Darlene Cohen used a similar method to overcome virtually paralyzing rheumatoid arthritis, as detailed in her book *Arthritis: Stop Suffering and Start Moving.*

☙ *Emotional and Physical Pain* ☙

Hard as it is to face, we often need to accept that emotions play a major part in pain. Back expert Dr. John Sarno, author of *The Mindbody Prescription*, believes that the body creates elaborate structures of pain to distract us from emotional pain that is worse than the physical. Sarno says that repressed emotions, usually anger, require physical symptoms to hide behind. Without such symptoms we would have to deal with the unacceptable feelings. Sarno has found evidence that the brain can work with the body to create actual physiologic problems. For example, the blood flow to a particular area will be reduced, causing pain due to oxygen deprivation.

Sarno treats back pain by insisting that his patients accept the emotional pain and deal with its causes. When our bodies convert the pain of living into physical pain, we tend to feel ashamed of ourselves, or we refuse to believe that our fear, anger, and hurt feelings relate to our pain. But it's nothing to be ashamed of; it's how our body/minds work. The body's decision to take on physical pain to distract us from crueler emotional suffering—feelings of failure, frustration, loneliness, abuse, etc.—is an attempt to preserve our lives and function. Such pain should be treated at the physical, emotional, and spiritual levels both professionally and with a large dose of the self-care measures in this book.

— *All Right As Is* —

For years, orthopedic surgeons told me my twisted spine was so weak I should avoid all vigorous exercise, at least until I had surgery. They had me thinking of myself as a cripple. Then I met an elderly osteopath named Joseph Kushner, a small, quiet man who worked by himself on the fourth floor of a run-down office building. He put me on his table, grabbed me behind the knees and neck, and bent me in several directions. Then he said, "Your back is all right. Do what you want."

To me, that is real healing. Those of us in the health professions should never forget the power of telling someone, "You are okay the way you are." Negative predictions or prognoses can become self-fulfilling curses. The reason it's so important to hear the words "You're all right" is because many of us think we are fragile, that some terrible breakdown is going to befall us at any moment. This is particularly hard for those with chronic illnesses that have unpredictable courses. Is my headache a sign of stroke? Does my stomachache mean my cancer has returned? Probably not. We need to check things out, but usually, if we trust our bodies and care for them, they will be all right.

☞ Respect Your Body

Can we learn to give our bodies some credit for the intelligence and effort they put into keeping us alive and functioning? Can we learn, as Darlene Cohen puts it, to live from the body's point of view? She says this means living a simple life, because the body mostly cares about rest, food, warmth, and comfort. She cautions against the life of the "hungry ghost," the mind that is never satisfied with what it is doing but is always planning the next thing or remembering the past. The hungry ghost starves itself by never really experiencing the moment. It is ghostlike because it is never in its body. The body does the opposite; its only interest is in being comfortable and healthy right now.

"The body's needs and the ego's needs are very different," says Cohen. "I only go into my ego's needs [e.g., success or productivity] when my body is enthusiastic [about it]. If my body has some restless energy, that's when I move into ego."

Easy for her to say; Cohen is a daily meditator, with thirty years' experience living in the moment. Most of us, though, can strive to pay more attention to the body. I get this experience with one of my MS symptoms: "restless legs," involuntary spasms that sometimes come on when I'm trying to sleep. This is a common MS problem—non-MSers get it as well—but I finally noticed that the spasms only come when I still have energy to do something that needs doing, such as writing. If I get up and do some work, then go back to bed when I'm really tired, the legs don't jump anymore, a good example of self-monitoring. When we respect our bodies enough to let them call some of the shots, we are on our way to more pleasurable, relaxed lives and better health.

⚊ *The Zen Master's Knees* ⚊

Can we really love ourselves and consider ourselves worthwhile without loving our bodies? Cohen worked with an elderly woman, a teacher of Japanese tea ceremony who had developed severe knee pain from long hours of kneeling in meditation. Cohen taught her a knee massage, and on a return visit she asked the client to demonstrate how she was doing the massage. Cohen says, "She began massaging, and she said to her knees, 'Oh, little knees, you have carried me up the stairs; you have held me in tea ceremony; you have taken me on hikes,' and then she said, 'now it's my turn; I'll take care of you.' And I thought, my God, if all middle-aged people felt that way: 'you've played tennis, you've been my slave all these years, and now it's my turn to care for you,' people would have a lot less suffering."

Most of us are a long way from that woman's loving attitude. When we think about our bodies at all, we are usually critical: too fat, too wrinkled, too ugly, too something, or not enough something else. Debbi Shapiro says we can learn to love our bodies, little by little. We start by looking at ourselves in the mirror. "Over time, we can start noticing the parts we really do love, even if there aren't many," Shapiro says.

Love includes compassion. Yes, we have imperfections, genetic weaknesses, minor or major disabilities, other pains and problems. Yes, we have gotten older; our bodies can no longer do everything they did years ago. And yes, we could have taken better care of ourselves, and yes, the world has been, and continues to be, hard on us in many ways. Our bodies, though, are doing the best they can, and they could use a little appreciation.

We need and deserve our own compassion. In spite of our mistakes, most of us have done pretty well—well enough, at least, to merit our own sympathy. It is never too late to forgive and care for ourselves. Even in severe or terminal illness our bodies may surprise us with how much they can improve, how much comfort, pleasure, and function they can still give. We just need to give them a little help.

If you're ready, turn to the next chapter to explore the positive dimensions of self-care, where we can take the lessons, skills, and attitudes illness teaches, all the losses and limitations, and use them to give our lives more beauty, meaning, grace, and health.

8

THE ART OF
GETTING WELL

*H*ERE'S MY FAVORITE ZEN STORY: A priest was going around winning many followers by performing spectacular miracles. One of these followers was walking with a Zen monk along a river. "Our master," said the disciple, "can stand on one side of the river and write the name of the Lord in letters of fire on the other side."

"My miracle," said the Zen guy, "is that when I'm thirsty, I drink, and when I'm tired, I rest."

No miracle beats living with simple grace, and overcoming long-term illness calls on our creative powers to help us live in peace with our bodies and with the world, like the monk by the river. Perhaps you didn't know you were an artist, but in the process of getting well, you may discover the ability to turn your life into an ongoing work of art, capable of fulfilling your potential, promoting your health, and enhancing the lives of others. The art of getting well is a martial art, a gentle form of self-defense against all the ways life can injure us or wear us down. Like a martial art, overcoming illness emphasizes rhythm, balance, and flexibility. These qualities can be applied in an enormous variety of ways, physically, mentally, and spiritually. The creative energy for this art comes from consciousness of our limits.

☞ Limits and Creativity

The great saxophonist John Coltrane sometimes played jazz that was completely free form. He produced amazing sounds that appeared to come directly from his soul, with little rhythmic or melodic structures the audience could discern. A few fans adored this music; some of them even started a church of Coltrane. Most, however, left this music alone; it was just too hard to understand.

When Coltrane played with trumpeter Miles Davis's group, however, the great saxman had to blend with the rhythms, melodies, and harmonies of other brilliant musicians. He strained against the limits imposed by Davis's music, but the creative tension of working within those limits inspired some of the best jazz ever recorded, music that has moved millions of listeners. This kind of story happens repeatedly in the arts, usually in a scenario where a star leaves a successful group for a solo career that bombs. It turns out he or she needed the limiting force of the group to create successfully. Limits bring out our creativity; without them, we tend to wander around dabbling in different things, accomplishing little that has meaning to others.

One of illness's little tricks is the way it shows us our limits. We always had them, but most of us preferred not to notice, choosing to live as if we were immortal and superhuman. That unrealistic attitude dissipates our creative energy. "Should I do this or that or this other thing? I want to do X, but I'll do something else. What difference does it make? I have the rest of my life, which is forever."

We don't have forever, though, and illness demonstrates that fact with symptoms, disabilities, and scary predictions of the future. It requires us, in the face of irrefutable evidence of our mortality, to change, adapt, grow, and create. Rob Mitchell tells how twelve years of living with AIDS has affected him:

> Being confronted with my own mortality...I learned about living with the end in sight, knowing that I have a finite amount of time here and embracing the power that comes from realizing you're not immortal. "I don't have forever to do the things I want to do, so I better do them now." That's the best thing I've learned.

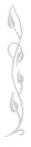

As we will see, Rob, like others who deal successfully with illness, responded creatively to the challenges of his condition. We all have the potential to respond in this way.

☙ A Balancing Act

If getting well is an art form, balance is the part the audience sees. The concept of balanced living is nothing new. It goes back to the Bible ("to everything, there is a season"), the wisdom of Lao Tzu in China, and the writings of Roman physician Galen. The serenity prayer—"Grant me the courage to change the things I can change, the serenity to accept what I cannot change, and the wisdom to know the difference"—is a prayer for balance.

As children, we were told about balanced eating and about developing physical balance. But living in harmony and peace involves a deeper sense of equilibrium. We must find the balance between our own needs and those of others, between living for the moment and for the (uncertain) future, between dependence and independence, and between acceptance, grief, anger, and constructive denial.

I think of getting well or living well with illness in terms of the Japanese tea ceremony, the ritual of focused concentration on the apparently simple task of making and serving tea. Moving slowly, fully experiencing each step, the practitioner of the tea ceremony turns the process into a meditation on grace and beauty. I doubt most of us will ever spend that much time making tea, but if we move at our own speed and find our balance, our lives can take on some of this measured beauty as well.

Warning: All that grace, beauty, and rhythm will fall apart if we try to follow others' tempo. I can walk pretty well at two miles per hour, but if I try to keep up with friends going faster, my gait will fall apart; I'll stumble around. The Chinese have a saying that no one can move gracefully when they hurry, so I don't hurry. Those friends just have to wait for me, and I have to accept falling behind if necessary.

A lot of people quit exercise programs after bad experiences with trying to keep up with the aerobics instructor. Others never even try; they look at Tiger Woods and say, "I can never play golf like that, so why bother?" As we age or become ill, we may hurt ourselves with comparisons

to younger, healthier bodies, including our own younger selves. The pain of such loss and frustration is real, and we must allow ourselves to feel it, but we should not let it stop us. Ideally, we use the pain to get out there and work on getting better. Finding balance is largely about finding our own speed, our own best ways to do the things we have been given to do, rather than comparing ourselves to some ideal or to those who are, or seem to be, doing better. Those others have their own problems.

How Long Is the Future?

When we face our mortality and limits, we tend to become more aware of how valuable each day, hour, and moment is. We tend to agree with Lindsay Lewis, a nurse with lupus, who remembers, "I used to try to be all things to all people. I was rearranging deck chairs on the *Titanic*. If I hadn't gotten sick I wouldn't have spent one minute living in the moment. I would have missed my whole life, not realizing that it is so precious."

We want to live in the moment, which is all we have, but we have no way of knowing how long that moment will be. That being the case, we have to find a balance between living for today and for the future. With creativity, we can do both. When Rob Mitchell was diagnosed with pneumocystis (PCP)—an AIDS complication that in those days usually meant less than two years to live, if you recovered at all—he had to decide how long "now" was going to be. What was he going to do with that time? He recalls:

> I was born in the SF Bay Area and have lived here my whole life. I thought, "I want to see the rest of the country." I had been waiting, trying to get someone to go with me. I had a nice motor home, but I couldn't find anyone who wanted to go. After the PCP, I took off.
>
> My grandfather had a little teardrop trailer, and I always remember him saying, "One of these days, one of these days. . . ." He died about ten years ago, and never even left the state with it. And I'm running along looking for other people's approval, and my dad said, "I don't want to see you sitting around here in ten years saying, "One of these days. . . ."
>
> What I learned is, if something is important to me, I need to be out there doing it. I also thought, though, I don't want to learn all this stuff and have it be wasted. Have it get stuck in my brain, which may at some point stop

functioning. So I took my computer with me and wrote these massive travel diaries and sent them out on the Net, e-mailed them to all my friends—what I'd seen, what I'd experienced, what it felt like. Hopefully, I'll turn it into a book, but anyway, it's out there.

Rob didn't abandon the future. He came back from his trip when he needed more support for his health. When the protease-inhibitor drugs came out, he started taking them, and he is now studying for a college degree as well as volunteering to counsel and teach others with AIDS. But the fact remains that he decided to take his trip—living as if now were all he had—and he is still alive, whereas nearly all his friends from the time he contracted AIDS are dead. In addition, people who have seen his travel diaries tell me they are very glad to have read them.

☙ Dependence vs. Independence

Like all the two-way balancing acts discussed in this chapter, dependence and independence are both necessary characteristics. All of us are dependent on others to a large degree and independent to a larger or smaller degree, but we generally want to stay close to a middle path. Different cultures and different situations call on us to veer more to one side of the line or the other. Being very young or very old, or having significant physical- or emotional-health problems or disabilities pushes us toward the dependency side, and that is all right. Being adolescent or having unfulfilled abilities, values, or desires squashed by a too-close family structure may call for more independence. That is okay, too.

A general rule is to keep doing what we can for ourselves if we don't compromise our health, safety, or quality of life in the process. But if we really can't read the numbers on our insulin syringe, we simply must get someone else to do it, or we must find ways to adapt (such as using syringes with bigger numbers). We don't want to act like the senior in the old joke who says, "My neck is too stiff to turn my head; my eyes are shot, my hands shake, I don't react like I used to, and sometimes I get confused. But, thank God, at least I've still got my driver's license!"

Creativity and the use of supporting aids can help us maintain independence. Some of us don't want to use a cane, walker, or wheelchair

because they make us feel dependent and embarrassed, like we've given up. Instead, we just don't go places we'd like to go. Which of those options is really giving up? There are catalogs full of great stuff to help people with various disabilities do almost anything. Sometimes it's not even new equipment we need, but rather a new attitude. As disability activist Susan Haight-Liotta says, "Disability doesn't mean giving up doing things. It means finding different ways to do them."

Finding different ways to do things is called problem solving; keep reading for some examples. The process involves brainstorming possibilities—by ourselves or with friends, family, or health professionals—then picking one and trying it out for a week or so to see if it works and then modifying it as necessary. If it doesn't work at all, pick another and try again.

Hundreds of tips, strategies, and techniques have been developed for getting things done with disabilities and/or reduced energy. Books with lists of helpful hints are given in the Resources section at the back of this book. Other advice is available from physical therapists, rehabilitation counselors, nurses, occupational therapists, support groups, and anyone who has limitations similar to your own.

Others and Ourselves

The balancing point between others and ourselves is hard to find. Some of us feel guilty for taking any time away from others. Others never think about anyone but themselves. Some cultures expect extreme devotion to family—that people place others' needs above personal needs—especially from women.

We reach balance in this aspect of life when we take all the time we need to maximize our health, without jeopardizing the health and safety of loved ones. We cannot take a two-day retreat in the country, no matter how much we feel like we need it, if it means leaving children alone in the apartment or spending the baby's immunization money. But when we skip our daily relaxation because Aunt Pauline wants a ride to the store for cat litter, we have gone too far the other way.

Sometimes balancing competing needs calls for creative solutions. Perhaps we want to get a massage. But it costs sixty dollars, money we've budgeted for our kids' Christmas presents. Possible solutions might include: bartering a service to the massage therapist instead of paying cash,

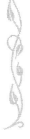

making something for the children instead of buying them gifts, or getting the money from somewhere else—perhaps by asking for help or using savings. An even better answer might be going to the local massage school and getting one for free from a student. Or, maybe we have a friend or relative who enjoys touching and could give us a decent rubbing.

A really important lesson is learning to let others live their own lives. We cannot afford to take on the problems of others who are capable of taking care of themselves. We can coach, advise, listen, and support, but they must make their own decisions and take the consequences. It's sometimes hard to apply this rule, especially with family, but we can save a lot of heartache on both sides by letting go.

Finding balance between visiting others and having time alone makes a big difference for me. Too much time with people, even with my wife, Aisha, can wear me out. I really treasure the days I can spend alone, but that's because I don't get them very often! For many of us, too much loneliness is the bigger problem, but for all of us, the key is finding the right balance, the mix that feels good to our bodies and spirits.

⌒Anger, Acceptance, Denial, Grief...

By now, most of us have heard of the stages of grief, identified by Dr. Elisabeth Kübler-Ross: denial, anger, bargaining, depression, and acceptance. Because they're called "stages," many of us hold the misconception that we go through the process in tidy steps—and then we're done with it. That may happen when we die, but most of the time we experience all these emotions simultaneously and repeatedly, and we face the task of finding balance between them.

With or without illness, a certain amount of denial is necessary for proper functioning. We may have a major health problem, but we don't want to think about it all the time. We need to face our mortality, but facing it constantly gets to be a drag. If we are facing a loss too great to bear all at once, some denial can keep us going until we are ready to handle it. Perhaps the saying "God never gives us a heavier burden than we can carry" really means "We only recognize as much of the truth as we can deal with."

Grief is also good, but not all the time. As discussed earlier in the book, crying and intensely feeling the loss and pain of our condition—

or of any loss—will enable us to get moving again. Feeling these feelings also allows us to fully experience the joy and beauty of life. I probably do some serious crying at least two or three times a month. That's what keeps me so annoyingly cheerful and positive the rest of the time. Life is full of sorrow and loss, so if we suppress sadness, our ability to feel anything will be dampened and eventually so will our ability to function. When dealing with an ongoing health condition (such as life), new losses will come and old losses will recur when we least expect them—and then we find ourselves needing to grieve again. It might even help to listen to a sad song or watch a sad movie occasionally, just to get the benefits of crying.

—— *Anger for Good and Ill* ——

Anger also plays a role in getting well, though too much of it can be deadly. If you have a chronic condition and have never gotten angry about it, you may still be in denial about your situation. Darlene Cohen, in *Finding a Joyful Life in the Heart of Pain*, talks about shattering a jam jar against the refrigerator when her arthritic fingers couldn't open it. She says her anger gives her the energy to do the exercises and other health practices she needs to get and stay well.

We all have reasons for anger. Perhaps we were raised in an angry environment, discrimination has limited our opportunities in life, or money problems keep us living in an unhealthy situation. Maybe we were born with some bad genes or raised with poor health habits. Or, perhaps we are angry with ourselves for not making smarter choices or with others who have treated us poorly. Rather than staying stuck so that our anger serves no purpose besides raising our blood pressure and destabilizing our hearts, how can we use our anger to help ourselves?

Both people who practice Chinese medicine and many psychologists think anger's function is to energize us to make a change in situations that hurt us or our loved ones. The trick is using our anger appropriately instead of letting it use us. If Darlene had thrown that jar at her husband's head, she would probably have been out of balance. If we get cut off on the highway, we can stew in anger, allowing rage to build as we think all kinds of destructive thoughts about the other driver. Doing that, though, hurts no one but ourselves, because there is nothing we can change (think of the

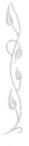

serenity prayer). The intended target isn't getting hurt; he's not even aware of our rage unless we commit an act of violence against him. In such a case, it's better to have a soothing thought ready, something like "He's probably under a lot of stress" or just to scream once and let it go.

Sally, a Healthier Living participant, demonstrated an effective use of anger after her rheumatologist gave her a series of drugs that caused stomach ulcers without helping her joint pain. He also told her that her spine was going to deteriorate, and nothing could be done about it. She finally said, "The hell with this." After checking with her pharmacist— to make sure it was safe to quit cold turkey—she stopped taking all her meds, stopped seeing the specialist (but continued seeing her personal physician), started taking supplements her husband found, and started flexibility and stress-reduction exercises. Now, fifteen years later, she still has some pain, but she's fully functional, stands tall, and enjoys an active, positive life.

Acceptance is where we want to be most of the time. Life feels better, uses less energy, and is easier to change when we accept it as it is. But we usually have to go through grief and anger to get to acceptance, and even then it is rarely a permanent state. It's something we need to work at. Sometimes, however, getting to acceptance is a goal we need to let go of temporarily. We need to give ourselves permission to feel our painful emotions. Sometimes we even need to spend a few hours, days, or weeks (depending on our condition) in denial. That doesn't mean "just one night on the town" for an alcoholic or an equivalent act of self-destruction. We have to take responsibility, but we can still allow ourselves a degree of emotional freedom.

☞ Self-Help or Self-Torture?

Self-help books (including this one) can make us feel overwhelmed because they are too full of things to do. Reading them, we wonder where we'll ever find the time to carry out all the wonderful prescriptions for our happiness. By this point, if you've read this book straight through, you've been told to get more pleasure, find more meaning, and spend more time and energy on self-care. Yet, we have limited time and energy, and most of us have other work to do.

Balance is the key element here, also. We tend to take an idea that sounds good, like exercise or relaxation, and treat it as an absolute requirement, a crucial responsibility, when it is just a tool. We encounter thirty ideas for things to do—and we believe we need to do them all and do them now. When you feel that way, stop! It is possible to gradually move into a healthier flow if we remember that no single role, job, relationship, health practice, or interest should dominate our entire life. Take it one thing at a time.

Rhythm Is Life

Pretend you're a car. Would you do better cruising down the freeway with your wheels maintaining a steady pace and a steady foot on your accelerator, or would you rather be stuck in stop-and-go city traffic, speeding up, slowing down, never getting a chance to run smoothly? Which way would you get better mileage? Which way would your engine last longer?

People depend on rhythm much more than cars do. Each body has its own rhythms—optimum patterns of wake and sleep, activity and rest—which many of us ignore. Living in a regular pattern allows us to flow along like a car on a freeway or like those elders who seem to go on and on, sustained by little except habit. This section advocates getting into a bit of a rut: learning and following cycles that are right for us, that feel good and use less energy. A recent study of people with MS found that disruption of their normal schedule was more likely to cause a relapse than was a major stressor such as death of a relative. Of course, we need variety too. The goal isn't to make every day exactly the same, but to live easily and regularly whatever we do.

— *Power of the Drum* —

Rhythm makes everything better. Beginning jugglers often struggle until someone turns on music. Music or a recorded drumbeat can help people with Parkinson's disease, multiple sclerosis, or stroke to walk better. Drumming has become a valued social activity in some senior centers because it promotes social interaction and improves functioning in people with

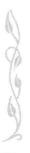

Alzheimer's disease and arthritis. Drumming and music therapy both have shown benefit for autistic and emotionally disturbed children.

Neurologist Oliver Sacks, who wrote *Awakenings*, says, "I regard music therapy as a tool of great power in many neurological disorders—Parkinson's and Alzheimer's—because of its unique capacity to organize or reorganize cerebral function when it has been damaged."

You can actually see this organizing effect on brainwaves, as demonstrated by EEG tests. Connie Tomaino, director of the music therapy department at Einstein Medical Hospital in New York, reports, "People who had irregular or weak background brain rhythms became more organized, and the rhythms became more pronounced and higher in frequency when more rhythmic music was played." The EEG improvements were often accompanied by functional improvement.

Music therapy has proven effective in all manner of psychological and physical conditions. According to Marc Ian Barasch and Caryle Hirshberg, authors of *Remarkable Recovery*, "In nearly all cultures, music and rhythm have been used as forces of healing.... Shamanic healing ceremonies almost invariably feature music and drumming." Usually shamanic drummers play at the tempo of the theta waves in our brains, the waves associated with imagination, dreaming, and creativity. In some cultures, the gods of healing are the same as the gods of music, as with the Greek god Apollo.

The benefits of music and rhythm should come as no surprise. Our bodies have their own flows: heart rhythms, four different brain-wave patterns, and muscle contractions. We all know the benefits of regular bowel (and bladder) function. The more rhythm we get in our lives, the easier things tend to go. We can play upbeat music when we are feeling fatigued, and gentler sounds when we need to relax. Rhythm means much more than music, though. It relates to the way we live.

— *Daily Practice* —

Bodies like to get up and go to bed at approximately the same times every day. Rotating shifts at work (especially the aptly named "graveyard shift") have been found to decrease life span and increase rates of illness. We want to find a way of life that will allow a reasonably regular schedule of sleeping. There will be special occasions, of course, but before and after these exceptional days we want to get back to normal. We also want to eat at fairly regular times.

I strongly recommend setting regular times for our health practices, whatever they are. I do stretching and meditation first thing in the morning, before anyone else knows I'm up. This plan works for a lot of people.

A wonderful health practice in much of the world is the siesta, usually an after-lunch nap at the hottest time of the day. In cooler climates, another time might be better. An after-work nap may fit best in most people's schedules. If a nap doesn't interest you or doesn't fit into your schedule, consider taking breaks between work and home responsibilities. A shower, a short walk, five minutes of focused breathing, reading the comics, or any kind of break helps us relax before facing the family or whatever awaits us.

It is good to schedule in time with our family, time for activities we love, and the other things we need to do. Don't forget to include some unscheduled time on your schedule! Life often happens in between the supposedly important events. Organizing your day is covered in the self-help section at the back of the book, but the main point is to create days we can live with, rather than wearing ourselves out scheduling a million activities. We all must follow our basic personal rhythm, our own activity/rest cycle.

— The Activity/Rest Cycle —

Remember the activity/pain cycle, where we push on until pain, fatigue, or some other symptom makes us stop? Even if we don't have major physical symptoms, we all have optimum periods for activity, and exceeding those periods will leave us feeling worse, sometimes for days. We want to convert to the activity/rest cycle, working, playing, and resting in the rhythm that fits our bodies' needs.

All of us tend to push our limits, but we need to save that behavior for times when something really good or important is at stake. Otherwise we wind up with worse symptoms and worsening disease processes. We tend to believe that we can't take a break because we have so much to do, but, in fact, as we get more fatigued our efficiency drops off. It is more effective to take breaks and come back refreshed.

Susan Haight-Liotta works and raises two children, despite diabetes and chronic pain. She has learned the importance of being flexible with her time. "Allowing yourself the ability to have bad days is a big thing," she says. "It's very hard, but it's a step that you have to take. It's okay if I'm in the middle of a task to go lie down for an hour to get my reserves back up. It's okay to push myself because I've got this deadline, even though I may pay for it tomorrow. It's like when you get out of high school and you go to college, you have new time-management skills that you have to learn."

How do we create and follow a workable activity/rest cycle? Since every body is different, the best way to get that information is by gauging ourselves. At what times of day or after how many minutes of different kinds of activity do we get tired, pained, irritable, depressed, or whatever our symptoms are? How much and what kind of rest or relaxation do we need to get back to full strength? Different kinds of activity can be fatiguing in different ways. We may need to lie down after housework, while the best recovery after tough mental work might be a walk.

NeelAnne Keith, a woman whose chronic fatigue syndrome has failed to dampen her positive attitude, recommends setting an alarm to remind us to take breaks. Once we learn how long a stretch of housework or reading or playing with the children is best for us, we can set an alarm for fifteen, thirty, or sixty minutes—or whatever is appropriate. When the alarm goes off, stop the activity and take the needed time to really rest, possibly including a relaxation exercise or a nap. It's okay to let the kids watch TV or to put the dishes off until later so we can get our rest. For more difficult demands, such as dealing with a confused elder or severely disabled child, we may have to get some help.

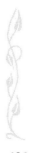

⟶ *Other Rhythms* ⟵

As recommended in Chapter 2, we should strongly consider taking a Sabbath day once a week. We may also want to move towards following the recommendation made by Chinese medicine: an annual pattern of living with the seasons. Chinese medicine says we should rest more in the cold and dark of the winter, avoid overheating in the summer, and consider starting some new activities in the spring, when the new plants are sprouting. Women may want to follow monthly routines based on the high- and low-energy days around their menstrual periods.

Able-Heartedness

Some final points on the art of getting well. When psychologist Joanne Lemaistre developed multiple sclerosis, she lost most of her ability to walk, as well as some other valued abilities. She persevered and wrote two books on living with chronic illness (what is it about MS that turns us all into writers)? In her book *Beyond Rage*, she develops the concept of "able-heartedness." "The truly handicapped of the world," she writes, "are those who suffer from emotional limitations that make it impossible to use the capacities and controls they possess. If you have a chronic disease, you need not be emotionally handicapped if you continually strive to become able-hearted. Able-heartedness is within the grasp of all of us."

— Humility —

If we don't want to be panicked by our limitations, especially our mortality, we need to recognize that the world doesn't really need us to do all its work. A wonderful feeling of peace comes over us when we realize life will go on just fine after we're gone, as it did for a million years before we got here. We can't do everything. The world doesn't revolve around us, and our "to do" list will still have things on it when we die. We might as well relax and heal.

The Green Triangle

This bit may sound preachy, but I'm going to say it anyway. I believe the amount of grace in our lives is often inversely proportional to the amount of driving we do. Ernest Callenbach, author of *Ecotopia*, promotes the concept of the "green triangle," with the points of the triangle being health, money, and the environment. Generally, living in ways that are better for the environment will save us money and improve our health. For example, drying clothes on the line instead of in a dryer saves on utility bills and conserves nonrenewable energy. It also gives us some good exercise and is easier on our clothes. Not driving is the prime example of this concept: you save a ton of money, eliminate what is likely the most stressful activity in your day, and help the environment. Try taking the bus, walking, or at least carpooling.

☞ "We're Dancing Inside Our Shells"

A lovely children's book titled *Clams Can't Sing*, by James Stevenson, tells the story of two clams who surprise their shore-dwelling neighbors by participating in the local talent show. They endure insults and doubts about their abilities but manage to come up with some kind of performance—blowing bubbles and making whooshing sounds, mostly. The crowd (of birds and crabs) loves it. At the end of the book, all the creatures are dancing, and a crab comes over and says, "Too bad clams can't dance." They reply, "We are. We're dancing inside our shells."

"I couldn't tell," says the crab. The clams answer, "That's not our fault!"

It's not our fault we have to live in these shells; everybody does, to some extent. But it is our responsibility to make our inner clam count, rather than be defined by the appearance of our outer shell. With that said, let us rejoin the world of the vertebrates and start developing our self-care plans!

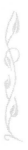

YOUR
SELF-CARE PLAN

A journey of a thousand miles begins with a single step—
or just by getting your behind out of bed.

Modified Chinese proverb

THIS CHAPTER OFFERS A MENU of possible self-care options for mind, body, and spirit, including ways to get moving, ways to slow down, help with healthy eating, plus mental and emotional self-treatments. A self-care plan, though, can include whatever you want: enjoying sunsets, helping others, reading the comics, finding new friends—whatever we can do on a regular basis to make life easier and happier. Remember, it's just a menu, not a prescription. If when you finish this book you're doing one more thing for yourself than you did before, you've succeeded.

No two self-care plans will be the same, because we all have different tastes, abilities, limitations, cultural backgrounds, and life situations. Our goals and our ways of reaching them will reflect where we come from, who we are, and what we like.

As Woody Allen said, "Eighty percent of life is showing up." It's essential to allow for reverses, bad times, and negative feelings; we must refuse to beat ourselves up for them and refuse to quit. When we experience anger or frustration, as we will, we can use those feelings as fuel for greater self-care. The more time, effort, and care we give ourselves, the better our lives are likely to get, so let's get started!

☙ Get Moving

With very few exceptions, such as immediately after a heart attack, exercise will help us wherever we are in our recovery. Bodies like to move. They were made to move, and they just feel better when they get some physical activity. The wonderful thing about exercise is that we can see results very rapidly. How can we believe we lack power to change our lives when we see that our muscles strengthen with weight training, that our legs or arms get more flexible with stretching, or that we can walk twice as far as we could when we started the program? Let's start with flexibility.

☙ *Yoga* ☙

For four thousand years, yoga has helped millions of people attain greater physical, emotional, and spiritual health. One of them, Eric Small, was a young adult when he developed severe multiple sclerosis, which progressed rapidly until he could barely walk. With little or no medical treatment available, he decided to try yoga. He had to crawl up two flights of stairs to the teacher's studio every day, but he persisted, and now, thirty-five years later, you would not know he had any kind of disability. He moves easily and looks great, although he still has MS symptoms.

Traditional yoga, or hatha yoga, is basically stretching; it consists of a collection of more than eighty asanas, or positions for the body. We focus on developing awareness of the body and of our breathing. We coordinate our movement with our breathing, go slowly, and pay attention to how different postures feel. The original intention of hatha yoga was to prepare the practitioner for meditation; accordingly, it affords the best results if it is treated as a practice in awareness rather than as work. More modern forms, such as Iyengar yoga and Bikram yoga, offer a more vigorous workout but lack the focus on awareness.

We have all seen pictures of the amazing postures yogis can attain, but such extreme flexibility is not the goal. In fact, most practitioners start

with very simple, quiet movements. Many of the postures are done in lying or sitting positions, which is good for many medical conditions. Teachers such as Eric Small have modified the traditional poses for people with disabilities. For example, we can use a wall or a chair for support in a standing pose or do certain stretches in a chair.

Tai Chi

Tai chi is not about preparing for meditation; it is a martial art. It is based on encouraging the flow of chi, or life energy, through the body (see Chapter 10). It focuses on graceful, flowing movements synchronized with breathing. It is difficult for beginners to imagine taking something so slow and graceful into combat, but the smooth motions of tai chi masters are incredibly powerful.

Chinese research shows that tai chi improves quality of life and health. Along with the exercises called qi gong, it is the favorite program for seniors in China and increasingly around the world. You can learn the basic movements from a book or tape or better yet from a live teacher. Virtually all tai chi is done standing, so people with major leg weakness, pain, or balance problems might prefer something else. On the other hand, tai chi is perfect for people with congestive heart failure since it involves little bending. It is not, strictly speaking, a program of stretching, so you may want to supplement it with other stretching exercises.

Plain Old Stretching

We don't really need a three-thousand-year-old Asian practice to stay healthy. Any program of stretching will help, if it is done with awareness of the body and attention to breathing. Some stretches can be performed anywhere and at any time. A ninety-two-year-old woman on my local bus does her foot and ankle stretches all the way to her destination. We can learn stretches from books, videos, magazine articles, physical therapists, and many other sources.

Those of us who can't move much due to muscle or nerve problems will benefit from having others help us stretch, in order to gently expand our range of motion. Here again, the goal is to pay attention and try to actively participate in the movements rather than just sitting passively

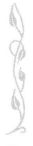

while someone else moves our limbs. Assisted stretching is gaining popularity in rehabilitation from strokes.

We all benefit from stretching as often as we can. Many like to stretch first thing in the morning, before even getting out of bed. Loosening our bodies makes getting up easier.

⬥ *Building Endurance* ⬥

Activity that speeds up the heart and lungs and raises body temperature is what most people think of as exercise. When done correctly, endurance—or aerobic—exercise helps on four levels. It feels good, increases energy, improves long-term health, and builds self-confidence. My local YMCA is full of people in their eighties who exercise regularly, with the energy and optimism most people in their forties wish they had.

Here are three tips to successful endurance exercise:

Get a partner, if appropriate. Some of us are perfectly happy exercising alone, but others find it easier to stick to a program if we have company. We don't want to let the other person down, and their companionship makes the experience more pleasurable. Those looking for an exercise friend may find one at the Y, mall, health club, or senior center. Be prepared, though. Sometimes our exercise partners can't or won't meet our schedule, so we need a backup plan, especially if the friend provides the transportation. Perhaps a neighborhood walk or a stationary-bike ride could replace the intended gym workout.

Incorporate pleasure or fun. If our program is walking or running, we can do it in a nice environment like a park or mall (assuming one is available). Mall walking is a great invention for those who live where it's too cold in the winter or too hot in the summer to exercise outdoors. Consider playing a sport with a ball or toy or playing mental games while exercising.

Learn your safety limits. We may want to clear your exercise programs with our doctors, though this is usually not required unless we plan to undertake a strenuous exercise program. We do need to know when we're doing too much. If we can't talk or sing, we need to slow down or stop. You should stop and rest immediately if you experience chest pain, or get help (and take your medicine) if it doesn't go away. Another indicator is "self-rated exertion," which means rating how hard we are working on a scale of zero to ten, with ten being the hardest we could possibly go. We want to stay between three and six, except for short bursts of effort. Some people take their pulse rates and compare them to target rates (which you may want to discuss with a doctor). It should take less than ten minutes to recover after exercise; if you have to take an hour nap, you have done too much.

⟶ *Walking and Running* ⟵

For those with good legs, walking is simple, cheap, and safe. Sometimes we don't need a regular program at all. Just park farther away from your destinations, walk instead of drive to the store, or take the stairs instead of the elevator.

For walking or running, it's especially important to get properly fitting shoes, preferably more than one pair. This is especially important for people with diabetes, who should not risk any pressure sores or scrapes to the foot. All exercise clothing should be comfortable.

How much exercise is enough? Most experts say 120 to 150 minutes a week is all we need. Few claim increased health benefits from going over 150 minutes weekly.

⟶ *"Sit and Be Fit"* ⟵

Those whose walking ability is limited can do aerobic exercises while sitting. "Band-leading" is one, vigorously waving our arms around to music, as if leading an orchestra. We can also do arm lifts, with or without weights. Some televised fitness shows include "sit and be fit" programs. "Sit and be fit" videotapes and books are also available, and one book worth looking at is Charlene Torkelson's *Get Fit While You Sit* (Hunter House Publishers, 1999).

➳ *Water Exercise* ➳

Some people have no pools or lakes nearby, but those who do have access to water enjoy a nice advantage. Water supports some of our weight, making it possible to do exercise we couldn't do on land. Water exercise creates much less impact on the knees and hips. Most YMCAs and health clubs offer a number of water-exercise programs—or we can just swim laps. Water temperature is an issue for some folks. People with arthritis and certain heart conditions want warm water, whereas people with MS need cooler temperatures. You may have to call around to find a pool with the right level of heat. As with any other exercise, start slow and listen to your body.

You may have access to a pool you didn't know about. Most colleges and some high schools have pools, and some make swim time available for members of the community, especially people with medical necessity. Some private clubs may offer scholarships or reduced rates for people with medical needs.

➳ *To Gym or Not to Gym?* ➳

Should we join a gym to exercise? Gyms have a lot of equipment, so they offer a variety of possible movement programs. Many also offer classes and trainers to help members exercise more effectively. Some provide a nice social environment, which can be an incentive to work out more often. On the down side, some of us don't want anyone else looking at us while we exercise, especially in shorts. We may perceive the gym crowd as much younger, healthier, prettier, or more upscale than we are. Not to mention the fact that joining costs money.

It is often possible to find a gym attended by people who look like the rest of us. We can visit several until we find one where we would feel comfortable exercising. If we want, we can exercise in baggy exercise clothing that hides our bodies. If we're concerned about expensive gym fees, some clubs, especially YMCAs and YWCAs, offer subsidized memberships for those who need them.

But joining a gym is never necessary. There are plenty of good exercise activities that don't require equipment and plenty of books and videos to tell us how to do them. Some exercise equipment, like stationary bikes, is available at thrift stores for as little as twenty dollars. If you do join a gym, make sure it's one that offers a month-by-month membership, without a large joining fee. Clubs that sell lifetime memberships are usually rip-offs.

Other resources for affordable exercise include community and senior centers, park and recreation departments, community colleges, hospitals, medical groups, and disease-specific organizations like the Arthritis Foundation.

Be aware that some fitness trainers at commercial gyms have little medical knowledge, so we still must use common sense. If you have a concern about any of the trainer's suggestions, check with your doctor. My sister-in-law was hospitalized several times for sickle-cell anemia because she allowed a personal trainer, apparently ignorant about sickle cell, to push her into overworking, which caused the disease to flare up.

— *Other Good Endurance Programs* —

Cycling is low impact, so it can be good for people with back, hip, knee, or foot problems. Riding a real bike has the advantage of taking us places and getting us out in the air. A stationary bike has the advantage that weather will never interfere with your ride, but the disadvantage of boredom. The scenery never changes on a stationary bike. Nature videos or simulated bike-ride videos can give the illusion of a ride through the country. In either case get a comfortable seat, or you won't be riding long.

Other exercise machines are available in gyms or for home use if we have the space and the money. Stair climbers, cross trainers, treadmills, rowing machines, and hand cycles (or ergometers) all work for different people. The last two, operated sitting down, may work for those with leg problems. We can even buy a set of pedals to put on the floor so we can work out in a chair or from the bed. Tip: Don't buy a machine until you've tried it out a few times. Exercise equipment makes lousy furniture, but that's all it is in many homes after the first couple of weeks.

What about aerobics classes? As I've mentioned, newcomers to aerobics may get discouraged and quit if they try to keep up with the rest of the class or with the instructor before they are ready. It is essential to find a class that moves at our own speed and/or to be ruthless about slowing down or stopping when our bodies tells us to. Good aerobics instructors will demonstrate low-impact or slower options throughout the class. Don't be shy; before you join the class, interview the instructor about her or his teaching style! Another good trick is to follow the music at half speed. That way you can enjoy the benefit of the rhythm without exceeding your limits.

Dance, with its added elements of creativity and fun, is a wonderful endurance builder, and it also provides social interaction. The same rules apply: If we get short of breath or have difficulty talking or singing along, we slow down or stop.

⟶ *The Benefits of Strength* ⟵

Flexibility is more important than strength, but strength makes life easier. Because my legs are weak from MS, it used to be difficult and exhausting to carry bags of groceries, but strengthening my upper body has made shopping and doing laundry a relative piece of cake. Strength training is great for depression, possibly because it makes us take huge breaths, kind of like sighing, which is one way our bodies release grief. Strengthening also stimulates endorphin release, and feeling our muscles get stronger or bigger lets us know we can make desired changes after all.

When using weights, start with very light ones, and don't be in any hurry to increase. If you suffer from a heart condition such as congestive heart failure, you especially need to be careful using weights. It is better to increase the number of repetitions we do and the number of times a week we do them before increasing the weight. We may not need actual weights; we can use cans of food or other household objects. In fact, we don't necessarily need any added weight at all; many exercises build strength by using the weight of the body itself, as in arm lifts or leg lifts.

☞ Meditation, Relaxation, and Prayer

If movement is king of health practices, learning to be still is queen. We need to take time for focused breathing, meditation, relaxation, visualization, prayer, or just sitting there. Quieting our minds and relaxing our

bodies will bring short- and long-term physical, mental, and spiritual benefits. Here are some specific breathing techniques:

Pursed-lip breathing—The most basic breathing exercise. Get comfortable in any position. Breathe in through the nose, then gently breathe out through the mouth, with lips pursed together like you're going to whistle. Don't push the air out; let it come out slowly and smoothly.

Abdominal breathing—This can also be done in any position, although lying down may be easiest. Place your hands over the abdomen just below the navel. Breathe into the abdomen so that your hands rise up with the inhalation and lower with the exhalation. Let the breath relax your lower back as well. Ten slow breaths done this way should feel wonderful. If you get dizzy, you're breathing too hard.

Alternate nostril breathing—A very relaxing yoga technique, the most relaxing thing I know. Place your thumb and forefinger on either side of the nose, as though you're going to pinch your nostrils closed. Breathe in slowly, then push the right nostril closed and breathe out slowly through the left. Breathe in through the left nostril, then switch nostrils by closing the left and opening the right. Breathe out and then in through the right, then switch to the left, and continue. Out, in, switch. Repeat five to ten times or more if desired. This only works if both nostrils are clear.

Three-part breathing—Lying down, start by breathing into the abdomen, then fill the lower chest, then the upper chest. Then breathe out smoothly. Take a couple of smooth breaths before repeating. You can do the same thing on the exhalation; breathe in fully, then let the air out in three stages: upper chest, lower chest, abdomen.

⚊ *Meditation* ⚊

Breathing exercises such as the ones described above are a good introduction to meditation, the process of gradually emptying and/or focusing the mind. When thoughts enter the mind during meditation, simply notice them and let them go. For beginning meditators, thoughts pour in.

Gradually—over months or years—they slow down. I recommend setting a timer (not a loud alarm, however) because it helps the beginning meditator avoid wondering, "Isn't the time up yet?" Even if we do end up mostly thinking instead of relaxing, spending time sitting quietly is good for us.

Meditation in a group seems more effective and powerful. It's easier to focus when others are doing the same. Some health-care providers, churches, and community centers now offer meditation groups, or there may be a meditation center near you. For meditating on your own, hundreds of meditation practices, written meditations, books, and tapes are available.

Prayer

Prayer is much like meditation, except with a formal religious or spiritual content. When we pray, we are acknowledging a higher power and putting ourselves at its service. I believe it's important to say prayers slowly, so that not only God hears them but we do too. I also believe it's important to say traditional prayers in a meditative way, so that they mean more than simply the repeating of words we heard in childhood. Creating heartfelt prayers of our own may be even better. Group prayer may have even more powerful effects than individual prayer.

Relaxation Programs

Dozens of relaxation programs are available, most of them on tape. They offer help for sleeping, reenergizing, or just calming down. One method you can follow with or without a tape is progressive muscle relaxation. This involves lying down or sitting comfortably, and alternately tensing then relaxing each part of the body. I prefer skipping the tensing phase; I just consciously relax each body part, starting with the feet, ankles, calves, and working up through all the body muscles.

Millions of people relax with tapes that play peaceful sounds (natural or musical) or provide guided visualizations. They all work well, and some are even available at public libraries. You'll probably find you need to change the tape every couple of weeks or so, because most of them get boring and lose some of their effectiveness with repeated listening.

☞ Mental Self-Care

The mind can kill us or make us well. Hundreds of studies have demonstrated these abilities. Here's one example: Japanese doctors rubbed children with an irritating plant to which they were all allergic. But the doctors told the kids the plant was something that would make them feel good. Few of the children developed rash or itching. Then the researchers treated the youths with a harmless plant, but told them it was the poisonous one. Nearly all of the children broke out in severe reactions. These itchy kids have a lesson to teach us: We want to think of life as something pleasant, not as poison ivy. Below are some ways to do so.

— *Negative into Positive* —

A valuable technique for developing healthy attitudes is positive self-talk, that is, replacing thoughts of fear or self-abuse with healthier statements. As discussed in Chapter 3, with motivation and practice we can change even our most painful and harmful beliefs. Set aside time each day or week to work on developing positive thoughts, writing them down and practicing them.

A related technique is affirmations: creating general positive statements such as, "Every day I'm getting better." It's a good idea to make them specific to our situation. When I feel like I'm taking on too many things, I affirm, "I do one thing at a time, and that is sufficient." For my MS, I say every day, "Little by little, my immune system is learning to leave my nerves alone" or sometimes simply, "I have faith in my body."

Do affirmations really help? Few studies on affirmations have been conducted, but I think they are very powerful—if we can believe them. However, trying to force ourselves to believe an affirmation that makes us say "You must be kidding" probably won't work.

Positive statements and affirmations work much better when we say them out loud, preferably in a firm, clear voice. It's an excellent idea to say them to ourselves in front of a mirror and perhaps even better to say them to others, like we mean them. Sharing positive thoughts with the world makes our intention clearer; we start to believe it, and maybe the world does, too. See the self-help section at the back of the book for an exercise to help you create affirmations that work for you.

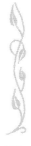

❧ *Visualization and Imagery* ❧

Employing the imagination is both relaxing and healing to the body. Athletes use imagery and visualization to train and to prepare for specific competitions. Literally hundreds of taped imagery experiences are available, including many for specific health problems.

We can also invent our own images. In interactive guided imagery (IGI), the tape or guide may simply ask, "Let an image arise for your symptom or problem" or "Let an image form that represents the healing of your illness." For my MS, I have visualized my white blood cells going to school, learning not to attack my nerves; the teacher at school was an old lymphocyte named Mary. I've created imaginary teams of knitters who repair my damaged nerve fibers. I believe these things help me, although few controlled studies exist of the effectiveness of such imagery. Depending on your condition, you might imagine your inflamed joints bathed in cool, healing liquid or your blocked breathing tubes or arteries opening up. You can visualize your immune system fighting cancer or infection. You might imagine positive goals—envisioning yourself running or dancing or whatever you are working toward.

Another good idea is to simply imagine ourselves in a safe, beautiful place where we can relax. We can imagine a place without pain or a place free from anxiety or stress. And, as discussed in Chapter 7, we can use our imagination to "listen to" our disease to get a better handle on it and on what we should do about it, or we can meet with a wise inner guide or inner healer.

❧ *Reframing* ❧

Reframing means looking at our situation from a different, more constructive angle. Most of us deal with plenty of pain, frustration, and loss throughout our lives. We can reduce our suffering by putting our situations into a different context. If, for example, our condition has rendered us much less athletic, we can compare ourselves with our younger, more energetic body and be miserable, focused on things we can no longer do. We can also focus on things we can still do and enjoy, remembering that many are worse off than we are. It is even possible to look at the positive side of loss. If we cannot work, for example, we can choose to give thanks for having time to rest.

If we regard a health problem as a curse, a punishment, or a death sentence, we will suffer more than someone who regards it as a manageable challenge or a learning experience. If we think someone in our lives is trying to make us miserable, we will probably have less stress if we reframe the situation by acknowledging that our tormentor has problems of his or her own. We still need to protect ourselves and find constructive ways of dealing with problematic people, but we don't have to increase our misery with pointless resentment.

⟶ *Expression of Feelings* ⟵

Dealing with hard feelings helps people get well. Unexpressed pain, anger, guilt, and fear are like heavy burdens that weigh down our bodies and minds. Consider writing in a journal or writing letters (probably not to be sent) to people who have mistreated us. We can talk to a friend or into a tape recorder. We can visit a clergyman or a psychotherapist. All of these measures have been shown to improve health and make people feel better about life.

⟶ *Mental Exercise* ⟵

Although not all psychologists agree, many believe that keeping our minds active helps prevent memory loss and mental deterioration. Mental activity can prevent boredom, provide fun, and distract us from unpleasant symptoms. We can do puzzles such as crosswords or play games of varying levels of difficulty. Or, we may want to read, think, or write about ideas or issues that interest us—the theory of relativity, maybe, or why cats play with string. Anything helps, as long as it keeps the mind active.

☞ Conscious Eating, Not Dieting

For many of us, healthy eating has been the struggle of our lives. Stopping nicotine is painful, but at least it's a one-step process. Dieting is a life-long national obsession. In the bookstores and on supermarket racks we see books and magazines with articles on diets, and even more ads appear on

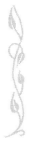

radio and TV. Almost none of them work, and many of them carry significant health risks, but people still buy them, because losing weight seems so difficult.

In HL class and in my practice, we discourage dieting. Dieting promotes a tense relationship with food that makes eating a high-stress experience—and that frame of mind doesn't do anyone any good. Instead, we want to tune in to our bodies and give them what they need. We want to eat a balance of grains, fruits, vegetables, and proteins, with a little fat and a few treats thrown in, but we can work towards that goal slowly. It's better to splurge once in a while on cake or ribs than to approach every meal as a battleground. We want to enjoy our food, not fight it.

Sugar, salt, and fat are not physically addictive, and they taste so good! We crave these substances because through most of human prehistory they were hard to get, and they were vital (in small amounts) to human health. We loved them because they were good for us. Now that we can get all the fat, salt, and sugar we want, it is still difficult to change our ancient cravings.

Healthier eating may involve giving up foods we grew up with and with which we associate the comforts of home, family, and childhood. Food often ties in with our cultural identity. "I am a person who eats a lot of meat with a lot of salt, just like my grandfather, father, and brothers—may they rest in peace—ate before me." We may not know how to cook or eat anything other than the foods we grew up with. We may anticipate, or actually have, problems finding or paying for healthier foods. Most communities, though, have at least one store that sells produce, grains, beans, and other healthy foods in bulk, which is usually cheaper.

Food carries an emotional wallop; most of us reach for chocolate, sugar, or fat when we are feeling down. Why shouldn't we, when we have been doing it since we were born? According to Geneen Roth, author of *Breaking Free from Compulsive Eating*, we may use food to substitute for love we didn't get from parents or use extra weight to keep the world away. We may feel, as a result of childhood abuse or neglect, that we are bad or unlovable, and we may overeat in order to focus those painful feelings on food instead of facing the deeper causes of our pain.

When we eat for emotional reasons or when we eat out of stress, we rarely even taste the comfort food. After the first bite, we just cram it in.

Instead, try the "make each bite count" technique. If we really slow down and taste the chocolate or chips or whatever, a couple of bites may satisfy us, instead of our needing the whole box. In fact, really tasting food, eating slowly and enjoying it, may be the most important diet tip of all.

We can also avoid comfort eating by the use of nonfood comfort measures, such as a hot bath, a shoulder rub (if a shoulder rubber is available), or a movie or other fun activity. Some people enjoy healthier comfort foods, such as dried fruit or nuts or a diet soda. Sometimes we can delay gratification by promising ourselves a reward in a few hours. By then, the craving may have worn off.

How Shall We Eat?

Food is not an enemy; it is a source of life. Our bodies can actually handle almost anything in proper amounts. Dangerous eating happens when we get too hungry or tired. That's when we reach for the bad stuff. We skip breakfast, and by ten A.M. we need a quick fix. We can prevent this scenario by eating regularly and carrying around healthy snacks, such as fruit, for when we begin to feel hungry, stressed, or tired. (Remember H.A.L.T.— Hungry, Angry, Lonely, Tired—the danger times for bad habits.) Here's another tip: Avoid temptation by keeping unhealthy foods out of the home and work environment. The best place to avoid temptation is in the store, not when the undesirable food is right next to your fork. If you work in a high-sugar setting, maybe you can maneuver the candy and cookies to a location you don't often visit.

If cooking healthy meals, or cooking at all, is a problem, we may be able to get help from others. If you live alone and don't like cooking for yourself, consider finding another single neighbor interested in sharing meals—you cook one; he or she cooks one. If we want to eat natural or low-sodium foods, cooking extra portions and freezing them for later can replace TV dinners and canned soups. Some of us need and qualify for having affordable meals delivered, as through the Meals on Wheels program.

Cookbooks may provide a ticket to new experiences. Try new foods once in a while; we might find something we love. Learning about new foods to eat and different types of cooking can turn healthy eating from punishment to adventure. Consult a nutritionist or dietitian or get

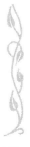

cookbooks (including free ones!) from an organization specializing in our condition, such as the American Heart Association.

~ *Supplements* ~

In my opinion, vitamin and mineral supplements can help most people, but not as much as some advocates claim. The effects are highly individualized. I had a client named Tess whose nineteen-month-old baby had severe asthma, for which the usual medications weren't helping. I suggested vitamin B-6, which *Prevention* magazine had reported as helping in preliminary studies. Although more recent research indicates B-6 doesn't confer much benefit in asthma, Tess's baby got well rapidly with it.

Most nutritionists say we can get the vitamins and minerals we need from eating a healthy, balanced diet. Many of us, of course, eat no such diet and may benefit from supplements for this reason. We may have to research which vitamins or minerals our diet is lacking or which are important for our particular condition. Some nutrients are shown by research to be good for most of us. These include the antioxidants, vitamins C and E, and the minerals zinc, selenium, and others; and the essential fatty acids, found in fish oil and several kinds of plant oils. Most women benefit from calcium and iron supplements, and some of us can use more magnesium. Talk with dietitians, doctors, naturopaths, friends, or the staff at the health-food store, or consult books or the Internet. Supplements can be expensive; experts vary on how much difference exists between expensive and cheaper brands. (See Chapter 10 for resources.)

⌒ Is That All There Is?

You may also want to plan how you will get more love, purpose, and pleasure in your life, as discussed in Chapters 2 and 5. It makes perfect sense to schedule time for fun, to make an action plan to look for romance, or to get counseling or read a self-help book to figure out what you want to do with your life. If helping others seems like a step you'd like to take, you can develop an action plan, maybe starting with as little as one phone call a week to a shut-in, to name one example.

The menu provided in this chapter covers some of the things we can do for ourselves. But most of us need more. There is a world of healing—and a great number of con artists—out there beyond the medical center. The last chapter covers finding and evaluating alternative, complementary, and mainstream therapies, and it addresses where all this self-care may lead.

10

BEYOND SELF-CARE

The truth is out there.

"The X-Files"

LTHOUGH WE DON'T WANT TO WASTE ENERGY, time, and money chasing illusory cures, we do want to keep our eyes and minds open. Sometimes partial or complete answers for our problems are out there, waiting for us to find them. At age forty-two my brother William developed a severe connective-tissue disease, diagnosed as tendonitis or perhaps psoriatic arthritis. Doctors weren't sure which it was, but as usual in such illnesses, the name didn't really matter because no effective treatment existed. When William's disease flared up, he couldn't open a door, button a shirt, or drive a car. His pain was constant and severe.

William saw several specialists and was put on steroids and hydroxychloroquine, an antimalarial drug that sometimes helps arthritis. It didn't do much for him. He went to acupuncturists, homeopaths, and several other kinds of healers. No soap. He even came to me. I advised him, probably wrongly, to cut back on beloved activities, such as bicycling and kayaking, that made his condition worse. He did cut back—he had to—but he still endured frequent, disabling flare-ups.

William researched dozens of possible remedies. He says, "Some were too far-fetched. If it seemed reasonable, I would try it. It's important to trust your doctor, but it's important to go beyond the doctor, too."

One day, another teacher at William's elementary school told him that his own arthritis had been the result of food allergies and had gone away when he stopped eating certain foods. Will went to his rheumatologist and suggested the food-allergy idea, but the specialist scoffed at him. Will said he was going to pursue it anyway, and his doctor helped by setting him up with an allergist. It turned out my brother had severe allergies to corn, wheat, and rice. Cutting these foods completely out of his diet has been a challenge—they're in almost everything we buy—but his symptoms have reduced by 90 percent. He still takes the medication, but he has his mobility and his comfort back.

Western medicine is the world's most powerful, but it is not the only source of healing. Self-care is critical, but we can't do everything ourselves. Scientific medicine offers effective treatments for many conditions, but there are large gaps in its understanding, whole categories of illnesses for which it has little to offer so far. Sometimes we have to think outside the box. This chapter touches on some of the less well-known sources of help—medical and nonmedical—that exist for nearly every physical and mental problem.

I am not suggesting we drop established treatments for some way-out alternative with no track record, and I definitely don't believe alternative treatments can take the place of self-care. However, when they are used as complementary therapies, along with self-care and appropriate medical treatment, I believe many of these practices can help.

We must employ an open but critical mind. I have seen some seemingly bizarre treatments work for friends and clients, but I also know of a fair number of quacks and con artists. There is no reason to give up, though. New medical and alternative ideas are appearing all the time, and old ones can still work even if they are no longer popular.

⌒ Evaluating Potential Treatments

How do we decide if a potential therapy is worth trying? First, does it make sense to us? If the rationale for the treatment is bizarre or seems unbelievable, we will probably not benefit from it. Second, does the therapy feel like a good fit? Author and cancer survivor Marc Barasch says the treatment, healer, and patient should be "congruent," meaning therapies should fit with our values, beliefs, and lifestyles. Although some have been healed at the shrine of Saint Bernadette at Lourdes, for example, very few non-Catholics have benefited. Some nonconformists might do better with alternative treatments they find for themselves, while strong believers in science might heal with the latest high-tech innovations.

In thinking about a potential new approach, we should evaluate it with some of the questions listed in Chapter 6. How good is the evidence backing it up? Have just a few people tried this treatment, or does it have a real track record? Just because a therapy lacks good supporting studies doesn't mean it's bogus or that we should stay away from it, but it is something to think about.

Multiple sclerosis has gathered a bewildering variety of alternative treatments. I have tried some I was drawn to: acupuncture, homeopathy, and certain supplements. The weirdest was bee-venom therapy, getting myself stung several times a day by bees. I gave it up after a week; it had too many side effects and gave me too much discomfort. Still, some people have reported great benefit from this treatment.

Like many chronic conditions, arthritis also has a long list of treatment approaches: everything from skin creams to herbal supplements, from chemotherapy to copper bracelets. We need to research as best we can the evidence for therapies that seem good to us. Support groups, the Internet, doctors, and health educators may be good resources. Be aware, though, that even totally discredited therapies—such as copper bracelets—work for some people.

✑ *Placebo Power* ✑

Such success may be due to the placebo effect, the activation of our unconscious self-care mechanisms through the power of belief. In some people the placebo effect is stronger than almost any medicine, while others hardly seem to experience the effect at all. If a particular treatment acts as a placebo for us, it can be just as valuable as a scientifically validated therapy. It's okay to experiment, as long as we do it safely—that is, by maintaining our regular treatments and self-monitoring.

Remember that the healer is sometimes as important as the method. Pay attention to the advice on choosing doctors and healers in Chapter 4. Don't settle for one who won't listen to you, explain what is going on, or explore options with you. Find someone you can like and trust. Suspect a practitioner who says he has to see you three times a week for the next year, "and then maybe we can taper off." Only rarely will we need expensive treatments so frequently. Be equally cautious about a treatment that claims "guaranteed success." No treatment works 100 percent of the time.

We might want to check on the credentials of alternative healers and doctors. How long have they been doing this? Where, or with whom, have they studied? What, specifically, do they claim they can do for us? What kinds of results have they had, and can they produce documentation of any of it? You might ask to speak with former or current clients to learn more about what you are getting into.

Alternative Therapies

Nature's Medicine

When my friend Rita was fifteen, she developed a bad case of Crohn's disease, an autoimmune disorder of the small intestine. When the Crohn's hit, usually in times of stress, Rita would endure terrible abdominal pains and profuse, bloody diarrhea, which forced her to miss school. At one point she missed a whole semester. Doctors had little to offer her besides steroid drugs, which gave partial, temporary relief while causing dangerous side effects. But Rita's mother found another doctor, who recommended a Brazilian herb called *pau d'arco* and a fatty acid called evening primrose oil (EPO). These supplements stopped her disease in its tracks, and she is now a successful fashion model.

While Rita's improvement is unusually dramatic for an herbal remedy, herbs are widely used in most of the world, and evidence for their use is as good as that for many chemical medicines. Because most of the studies come from Europe, American medical sources may be unaware of them. Some herbs, such as St. John's wort for depression, echinacea for colds and flu, and saw palmetto for the prostate gland, have gained wide (though far from universal) acceptance in the United States, and many others are sometimes effective.

159

My son Sekani lived with strep throat that hit him every single month when he was five years old. He would take two weeks of penicillin or some other antibiotic and feel better. A few days after the medicine was finished, the fever and sore throat would return. We finally took him to an herbalist, who said Sekani's immune system was underdeveloped and needed stimulation. He prescribed hot spices such as cayenne and cumin, which we faithfully put into small capsules and which our brave little son swallowed twice a day for four weeks. After that, his strep throat never returned.

☙ *Problems with Herbs* ☙

Since they are not classified as food or as drugs, herbal medicines are not regulated by any government agency. It is therefore hard to be sure about their claims of effectiveness or even whether the bottle actually contains the herbs listed on the label. Even when the real herb is present, it's hard to know how strong it is; strength can vary with the location or season in which the plant was harvested. We need to buy from a reputable company. Sometimes the staff members of health-food stores know which companies are reliable; sometimes they don't know. Internet companies can be even harder to check out.

General Nutrition Center (GNC) has a reputation for good quality control; they test their herbal products with sophisticated equipment to make sure they're the real thing. Some companies—including Nowfoods, makers of Now brand supplements—pay to have their herbs tested by stores who sell them. The herb and supplement industry in the United States and some other countries have started certifying companies for GMP (good manufacturing practices). For Chinese herbs, the California Association of Acupuncture and Oriental Medicine can provide information about the reliability of different brands; call them toll free at (800) 477-4564. The website www.supplementwatch.com, created and run by scientists, provides all kinds of information on various manufacturers and retailers.

Claims by the medical establishment about the dangers of herbs are generally overstated and somewhat misleading, considering the side effects of the mainstream medicines they advocate as safer. Still, significant risks exist with some herbs. Anything strong enough to do good can also do harm. Ephedrine, also known as ephedra or ma huang, is a stimulant that

can be too much for people with weak hearts; it has also caused some strokes and psychotic reactions. Some Chinese imports and Western preparations, including diet pills, often contain this herb. Some herbs interact badly with Western medicines. There is some evidence, for example, that St. John's wort reduces the blood levels of some drugs and increases the effects of others. We should inform ourselves of potential side effects and let our doctors and pharmacists know about herbs we are taking.

⟞ *Acupuncture and Chinese Medicine* ⟝

Chinese medicine is one of the oldest healing systems. It includes herbal medicines, exercises, and emotional balance, as well as acupuncture, the art of sticking needles in people. The theory behind acupuncture deals with the flow of chi, the life energy that runs through our bodies. We get chi from food, from breath, from sunshine, and from the Earth beneath our feet. Our chi must be balanced and unblocked for us to be healthy. The needles, herbs, exercises, diet, and meditations strive to balance chi.

Western science has never detected chi with any measuring device, nor can it be explained in terms of accepted physics, yet it is recognized in India as prana, in Japan as ki, in Polynesia as mana, and in many other cultures. If it does not exist, then believing in a fantasy has cured millions of people, but if it does exist, why can't we detect it? I am pragmatic; if this energy-based medicine works, I choose to believe in it.

So how well does it work? I know a lot of acupuncturists who tell me that the needles are particularly effective for pain conditions and problems with the female reproductive system, among other things. On the other hand, I've never heard of acupuncture doing much for people with MS—I've had three courses of it myself—or with many other autoimmune conditions. Still, some autoimmune patients say they have derived benefit. You have to decide for yourself on a case-by-case basis.

⟞ *Bodywork* ⟝

Healing with the hands is probably the oldest treatment of all. There are too many kinds of so-called bodywork to describe here, and they can all

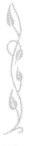

be good. Many are classified as massage therapies. The dozens of massage forms include Asian practices like shiatsu, a rhythmic massage, and acupressure, using fingers instead of needles on the acupuncture points. There are European practices such as Swedish massage, with firm pressure and long strokes. African and American peoples have developed massage styles, and many massage therapists use some combination of practices they have learned throughout their careers.

Massage by itself will rarely heal a significant health problem, but it can relax us, give us pleasure, and help us get in touch with our bodies. Sometimes it can even do more: relieve pain, bring more energy, free up restricted joints, help us move more easily. Studies have found that massage can reduce frequency of migraine headaches, asthma attacks in children, severity of back pain, and the chances of premature delivery by pregnant women.

Other forms of bodywork employed with massage or separately include craniosacral, the gentle manipulation of the skull bones, and rolfing, deep tissue work known for being rather painful and that works with ligaments, tendons, and fascia to actually change body structure.

⸺ *Nonmassage Bodywork* ⸺

Chiropractic is based on a system developed by D. D. Palmer in 1895. Palmer believed that most illness is caused by displacements of the spinal vertebrae, called subluxations. Chiropractors attempt to heal by adjusting the spinal bones back into place. Their license allows them to recommend herbs, exercises, and other treatments besides their trademark spinal manipulations, so if you find one who seems like a good fit, he or she may work well for you.

Osteopaths emphasize manipulation of the body to create better structure. They are also allowed to prescribe medicines in most states, so they can do much of what an M.D. can do. The focus in osteopathy, however, is on bodywork. Osteopaths have helped me and many others, but again, check out the individual practitioner you're considering working with.

━ *Movement Therapies* ━

Awareness Through Movement (ATM) was developed by Moshe Feldenkrais, whose central idea states that by learning more effective ways to move, our bodies reprogram themselves for greater comfort and health. ATM includes lying, sitting, and standing movements. It mostly emphasizes small and slow movements, performed with great attention to how they feel. ATM literally teaches new ways to sit, stand, walk, or even lie down. Small differences in position can make big differences in function.

ATM can be learned from a book or tape, but because each person's ideal movement pattern is different, it can be helpful to have a teacher. Feldenkrais classes, held at community centers, health facilities, or YMCAs, may be more affordable than private lessons. Once we have developed a personal ATM program, we can practice it on our own.

Another movement therapy, much recommended by dancers and other performers, is the Alexander technique, developed in the late nineteenth century. Like Feldenkrais, Alexander involves noticing movements and learning easier, more relaxed ways to perform normal activities.

━ *Psychotherapy* ━

Psychological problems can cause physical problems and vice versa. Our bodies react to negative thoughts and emotions, and any significant illness puts us at risk for anxiety or depression. Psychotherapy can often help. Good therapists help us deal with self-esteem issues, communication and relationship problems, and fear of change. They help us work through past injuries and psychic pain. Improvement in these areas will help us feel better and probably improve future health.

On the other hand, thousands of people go through extensive therapy without receiving much benefit. Talk therapy has the disadvantage of relying on the verbal mind, which resists change and is fully programmed with defenses against painful feelings. If we opt for psychotherapy, we should be ready to work. We will need to think about the issues between sessions, pay attention to our dreams, and notice and report any new feelings and thoughts that come up.

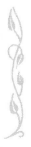

One issue to consider when choosing a therapist or type of therapy is whether we want to explore the deep causes of some painful pattern or whether we simply want to change it. Some therapies, such as brief solutions-oriented therapy, narrative therapy, and cognitive behavioral therapy, try to move clients out of bad places by focusing on our strengths. These therapies have the advantage of being faster, more positive, and often less painful. The disadvantage is that the problem may come up again later in another form. We should clarify your goals with our therapist so we can work toward them together.

Professional therapists include psychiatrists, psychologists, social workers, and, in some states, marriage and family therapists. Clergy, nurses, peer counselors, coaches, and others can also provide counseling. Some studies have found that, among licensed therapists, the level of academic preparation has little impact on treatment results; that is, an M.D. is usually no better than a master's-level social worker. However, only M.D.s can prescribe medications.

Most health plans pay for some psychotherapy, but they often encourage the use of medications, which are cheaper than therapy. Psychiatric meds can be helpful for many, especially in the short run, but they won't always help us change our lives. They help us cope, which is important, but they may not be enough for us to get well.

Less traditional forms of psychotherapy, currently gaining popularity but still very controversial, include Eye Movement Desensitization and Reprocessing (EMDR), which seems effective for problems related to trauma, and Emotional Freedom Technique (EFT) or Thought Field Therapy (TFT). EMDR has the client perform rapid eye movements while remembering traumatic events, which somehow seems to enable us to get a better handle on the emotions arising from the trauma. EFT and TFT are forms of "energy psychology," employing the acupuncture points or "energy flows" in the body by tapping or passing hands over various parts. It all may sound a little weird, but therapists and doctors for whom I have great respect say they are getting terrific results with these new methods.

⸺ *Naturopathy* ⸺

A naturopath is a doctor—with or without an M.D. degree—who emphasizes natural remedies, frequently herbs, in his or her practice. A huge
range of people call themselves naturopaths, from the highly educated
and skilled to those who took a few correspondence courses after high
school. A good one—as determined by the criteria listed above for choosing a healer—can provide excellent healing assistance, but check her or
his credentials carefully.

⸺ *Reiki and Energy Work* ⸺

Reiki, like qi gong, works with the life energy. Like acupuncture, it attempts
to enhance and strengthen the chi or ki, using the thought and intention of the practitioner to direct the energy flow, but it usually doesn't
involve touching the patient's body at all. Begun by Dr. Mikao Usui in
early twentieth-century Japan, reiki has spread rapidly in recent years. It
is gentle, safe, and relaxing. Some people report great benefits; others
say they noticed no effect of any kind. Scientific research on the effectiveness of reiki is being carried out as you read this.

Therapeutic touch is another energy technique, popularized by
Dolores Krieger in the '60s and '70s and mostly practiced by nurses. In this
method, the healer moves her hands near the recipient's body and
"smooths out," or unblocks, the energy problems she finds there. Many
other forms of energy work exist as well. Documentation of effectiveness
for these modalities is sketchy at best, according to Barrie Cassileth, a pro-
fessor and acknowledged expert on alternative medicine. They can't hurt,
though, and many find them useful as complements to more conventional
treatment.

⸺ *Faith Healing and Shamans* ⸺

I can't recommend particular faith healers, but I have known people who
claimed to have been cured. The recipient doesn't necessarily have to
believe in the healer's religion, but it helps. Whether the mechanism is
psychological, whether divine intervention is involved, or whether some

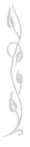

as yet undiscovered energy is at play, the cure rate seems quite low. But it does happen. One case, reported in the *Journal of the American Medical Association,* involved a twenty-eight-year-old woman with advanced lupus and thyroid disease. The usual medications were failing completely. She went home to the Philippines and two weeks later came back cured. She said her village witch doctor had removed a curse placed on her by a former suitor. The mechanism for her remission, which continued during years of follow-up, is unknown.

Prayer groups and healing circles get together and pray for the recovery of others. If you want to be prayed for, it may be possible to find such groups through churches, in newspaper classified ads, or on the Internet.

Shamans are individuals, mostly from tribal cultures, with great personal power or charisma. Often they are chosen in childhood for a life of healing through connection with the spirit world. They use music, herbs, and other methods to induce an altered mental state in themselves, the patient, or both. Then the spirits are invited to do the healing. One thing true faith healers and shamans have in common, according to anthropologist and shaman Dr. Hank Wesselman, is that they don't charge for their services. The recipient is expected to make a donation, but not necessarily in the form of money.

⚊ *Homeopathy* ⚊

Homeopathy, widely popular in Europe, is based on the Law of Similars, the idea that "like cures like." It was developed by Samuel Hahnemann (1755–1843) and has spread throughout the world. The patient is treated with a minimal dose of some substance that would in stronger doses cause the same symptoms as the patient's disease causes. Although homeopathic remedies are available over the counter, the basic concept is to treat the whole person, not just the symptom, so it may be difficult to know what to buy without first consulting a homeopathic practitioner. To me, the best thing about homeopathy is that the medicines are so diluted they cannot possibly cause any harmful side effects. My own homeopathic treatment neither helped nor hurt me.

⟶ *Extra-Strength Placebos Sold Here* ⟶

Many more therapies are vying for your attention and money. Many, even those with no scientific backing whatsoever, have helped thousands. One friend with a chronic problem went to a healer in a small town. This healer, who enjoyed a big local reputation, hooked my friend up to some strange electrical device, got some "readings," and prescribed "Syrup of Black Draught," an old-time laxative, which, on the surface, had nothing to do with his problem. He used the syrup, and his symptoms went away in a few weeks. Was this the placebo effect or an unknown benefit of the Black Draught? My friend does not care; his problem disappeared. If a therapy or a practitioner makes sense to us and passes the evaluation criteria listed above, they may well help us, even if their science is shaky and they seem a little strange. The same applies to new medical treatments, if they seem reasonable. Just be careful; research any treatment before you put your body and money on the line.

⟼ Checkups

Having one condition doesn't make us less likely to develop another. Having hypertension doesn't protect against cancer or arthritis against heart disease. Self-care for existing problems, as described in this book, will decrease our chances of developing new conditions, but it certainly doesn't guarantee anything. So it's important to get regular checkups for things like blood pressure, colon cancer, breast cancer, and diabetes, as recommended in medical guidelines. We need to do our breast or testicular self-exams and to brush and floss our teeth. Let's aim to live long, healthy, happy lives without spending much of them in the hospital.

⟼ What to Do After We're Perfect

Why are we going to all this trouble? After all, we won't live forever, even with the best healers and self-care in the world. We will still endure our share of pain and loss, sometimes more than our share. These statements are all true. But remember, being born is a death sentence; what counts is what

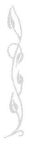

we do with the time we have. By taking care of ourselves, by optimizing our health, we get to participate fully in the good things that life provides. We get to benefit the people around us and possibly wider circles as well. We get to appreciate the gifts of life, not just endure the struggles.

I see self-care as a spiritual path. When we start out, we may be struggling to keep our head above water in a sea of frightening changes. However, as with a religion or a martial art, we grow stronger and clearer the more we practice. Learning to live in our bodies connects us to the great life force of Mother Earth, of which we are a part. Over time, self-care leads us not only to better health but also to more awareness and higher states of consciousness.

But, as the Buddhists say, the path does not end when enlightenment is reached. We can take what we have learned and make the world a better place with our presence, and this, too, will make us healthier and stronger. This journey may end with death, or it may continue, but it can always be fascinating and rewarding. I wish you the best on your journey, and I hope we meet someday along our paths.

SELF-HELP

☙Action Plans

*T*HIS EXERCISE BREAKS DOWN LARGER GOALS, such as "get more exercise," into specific steps, thereby increasing the likelihood we'll achieve our goals.

Write down the days of the week on separate lines. At the top, write down what you want to do (e.g., "walk"); when you will do it ("immediately after supper"); how long you will do it or how far you will go ("twenty minutes" or "one mile"); and any more details you wish to add, such as where or with whom you'll do it ("around the high school track, with Mary if she's available"). (See Chapter 3 for more examples.)

Write down your confidence level, on a scale of one to ten, that you will accomplish the whole plan: ten = "I'm absolutely sure I'll do it"; one = "I'm just kidding myself. There's no way." Your confidence level needs to be at seven or above. If it's lower, consider making the plan easier, or else identify the barriers you think will get in the way and come up with a solution that gets your confidence up to seven. Ask for help if necessary—with brainstorming for additional ideas or with more concrete tasks, such as child care or housework.

Next to the days of the week, check off whether or not you carried out the plan that day, and make any other comments (e.g., "raining too hard," "doctor's appointment"). If you planned, say, to call your mother after dinner twice this week and to talk for ten minutes, you could check off the days you called. Keeping the log handy will remind you to carry out the action.

☞ Affirmations

Affirmations are positive, believable statements that we make to ourselves or to others. They replace the negative thoughts many of us habitually express and believe. They may also help us program our bodies and minds for healthier functioning.

Many books of prescripted affirmations are available, but I question the value of some of them. Statements such as "My life is unfolding in perfection and beauty" or "Every day in every way, I'm getting better and better" often don't hold much meaning for our specific lives, nor are they believable, except to the most positive of us. Here is an exercise for coming up with useful, believable affirmations of your own:

1. Write down one of the painful, negative thoughts you would like to change (e.g., "I'm too busy to take care of myself"). It may take some work to even identify negative thoughts. When you're feeling bad—angry, depressed, sad, inadequate, afraid—you can probably get in touch with a negative thought behind the feeling.

2. Reverse the negative statement into a positive one, something that you want and that you can believe, stated in the present tense. For example, "I'm too tense" could be changed to "I am relaxed and centered." However, it needs to be a statement you can believe. If it's not, keep working until you come up with one you *can* believe, maybe "I am able to relax."

3. When you've come up with an affirmation that feels right for you, say it frequently. Say it aloud. Especially use it when negative thoughts or feelings come up. Sooner than you think, you will have replaced

them with positive thoughts. After learning to accept a mild positive, you may find you can strengthen it (e.g., change "I can relax" to "I am relaxed").

Important: Keep in mind that affirmations only work to change your own feelings, thoughts, and behaviors, not those of other people. It won't do any good to affirm that your husband is going to lose weight or start helping more with housework. You can affirm, however, that you will be more assertive about asking him to help.

☞Anger Reduction

Keep an "anger log." Write down each time you become angry: the time, the circumstances, how long you stayed angry, and how angry you got on a scale of one to ten. You might begin to see a pattern of what makes you angry and when. You may note, for example, that you become angry in late afternoon, when you might be tired and/or hungry or when your father calls to discuss your career. If you can't avoid the anger-inducing situations, perhaps you can prepare for them.

Learn to identify your anger-arousing thoughts, such as "It's not fair"; "It's their fault"; "You're not treating me right." Change them to calming thoughts, such as "She's probably having a bad day"; "Bad things happen to everyone"; "Maybe he couldn't help it"; or "I can't fight every battle."

If anger persists, use the energy generated by your anger for self-care. Exercise, do some deep breathing, laugh at the situation, or distract yourself with an activity you like.

Other anger-reducing behaviors include walking away, assertively standing up for your rights without getting angry, thinking about your part in the situation, and, especially, taking steps to solve the problem behind the anger. Continue practicing these new behaviors and keeping the anger log; you may note the frequency, severity, or duration of anger episodes decreasing.

✐Appreciating Our Bodies

Take a few weeks for this exercise.

1. Once or twice a day, look at yourself in the mirror and say, "I love you." If you can't admit to loving yourself, try, "I accept you the way you are" or "I appreciate you" or some other positive statement. You may want to start slowly, not even looking yourself in the eye at first. Work up to it; try saying your positive sentence louder and with more feeling. Keep saying it until you mean it.

2. Now remove a piece or two of clothing. Try saying "I love you" when you can actually see more of your body. When you can do this, try looking at various parts of your body, especially ones you aren't happy with, and saying those three words (or your alternate positive statement). Work up to being able to say "I love you" to yourself when you're naked.

3. Try imagining parts of you that you can't see, such as internal organs, especially those that are not doing well in your current state of health. Think about what they do for you, how hard they work, how much pain they go through. Say, "I love you" (or your alternative) to them. Again, keep repeating this step until you believe it.

This exercise is tough. We have all absorbed so many negative attitudes about our bodies that it is hard to feel positive about them, but many authorities, such as Dr. Bernie Siegel, say self-love is the critical factor in getting well.

✐Appreciation

Somewhere near the end of the day, write down five things you appreciated about the day. Anything could make your list, from the taste of the cinnamon toast at breakfast to a compliment someone gave you to a peace treaty in Mongolia. To make this exercise more powerful, keep it in mind as you go through the day. When you bite into a tasty sandwich or hear a nice birdsong, take time to savor it and add it to your list of five. Give thanks for these things.

List as many people as you can who have made a positive contribution to your life, from babyhood to the present day. These can include your most intimate family members or people you have never met, like a singer whose music you love. Reviewing the list reminds us of the gifts we have received and continue to receive on a daily basis. A follow-up is to write a thank-you letter to someone on the list, living or dead, telling him or her what he or she has meant in our lives.

Here's a family exercise: Once a week or more, at dinner or another family gathering, take turns saying one thing you appreciate about each person at the table, including yourself. It may be hard to get the kids into this at first, but it gets easier, and it helps the whole family feel better about themselves and each other.

⏖ Assertiveness

For some reason, assertiveness isn't the hot topic it used to be, but it's still a great need if we want to get well. Here are a couple of practice exercises. Most of them work better with a partner so that you can "role play" the assertive behaviors.

Saying no—Make a list of four things you would like to say no to. These could be dates, work assignments, plans for fixing up the house, or whatever. Then ask yourself what would happen if you said no. Maybe ask a trusted friend if your concerns are realistic.

Pick one thing off your list, and go ahead and say no. See if any of the terrible things you'd dreaded as a result of saying no come to pass.

Practice how you will say no to a request you don't want to accept, without apologizing. Your language should be simple and straightforward (e.g., "I know we usually get together for lunch on Fridays, but I need to rest this week. We can reschedule for next week.").

Difficult situations—Plan ahead how you will deal with some difficult conversation in an assertive way. Think of what you will say, how you will say it, what your body language will be. Practice. Assertiveness teachers say our tone of voice, volume, and posture say as much as the words do.

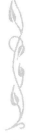

Here are three practice (role-play) situations. Alternatively, you can substitute your own. Formulate "I" messages in response to each other. Remember the three parts of the assertive "I" message: "I feel X, when you Y, because it affects me in Z way."

> One of your supervisors at work is constantly riding you. When you get upset by his actions, he switches to, "Can't you take a joke?"

> You feel a family member has been very unaccepting of your needs (time to exercise, time to relax, affection, communication, etc.). Confront him or her about your feelings.

> Your nosy uncle calls to tell you he will arrive next week to stay with you for three weeks.

Asking for help—Think of three things you sometimes could use help with. (Make them things you don't absolutely need, but could benefit from.) Examples might include washing dishes, getting a ride to the hospital in a nonemergency situation, finding a job, having a designated representative for medical decisions. Who would you ask for help and what would you say? Remember, keep it simple, be as specific as possible, and don't apologize. When you're ready, actually ask for something that you normally don't ask for, and see what happens.

Giving compliments—Practice giving one honest compliment a day, one that expresses your true feelings. Build up to three a day, or more.

⌒ Forgiveness

Complete the following two affirmations. Be easy on yourself if you can't honestly forgive yourself or others right away. Remind yourself that forgiveness is usually a process; rarely is it a one-time event we accomplish simply by mouthing the words "I forgive." Thinking about these statements may bring up issues that you need to explore more deeply by writing in your journal or sharing with a trusted friend or professional counselor.

I fully forgive myself for _____.

I fully forgive _____
for not meeting my expectations and for not being the person I wanted him or her to be.

For grudges against those who have done you serious harm, Dr. Fred Luskin, author of *Forgive for Good*, suggests the following program:

> Understand that your goal in forgiving is to feel better and commit to that goal.
>
> Recognize that your distress comes more from your reaction to what was done than from whatever actually happened.
>
> When the angry feelings start to come up, focus on your breathing, and think a prechosen positive thought.
>
> Stop expecting other people to change; find other ways to get your needs met.
>
> Concentrate on living the best life you can, on finding the beauty and love that are still there for you, in spite of the injuries you've suffered. (I sometimes say that when you're happier than the person who hurt you, you've won. But that may not be spiritually correct.)

☞ Priorities

In her book *Take Time for Your Life*, personal coach Cheryl Richardson suggests recording how we spend our time for a week. Make a chart and see where the time actually goes. The things that take most of our time are our actual priorities, whether we like them or not.

Once we have this information, we can then make a new list of the things that truly matter to us—the priorities we really want—and see how to reschedule our time to make more room for them. To help people figure out what they really want, Coach Richardson asks questions like these: What's most important to you at this time in your life? Where would you

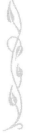

like to spend more of your time? If you could do anything you wanted, without restriction, what would it be?

Look at the ideas these questions generate, and create a priority list that reflects what is really important to you (your "Absolute Yes List"). Then figure out ways to make time for those priorities. Doing so will require creativity, cutting back on other things, and using assertiveness to say no to things that really aren't priorities.

Psychotherapist Sara Doudna suggests going through each aspect of our lives—clothes, activities, household maintenance, even people—and asking ourselves, "Does this cost me more energy than I get from it?" If it does, consider changing it or getting rid of it.

☙ Purpose

In training to work with dying patients in hospice care, we practiced writing our own obituary.

Write your obituary twice—once as you would like it to appear and once as you think it would actually read if you died tomorrow. If there is a large discrepancy between what you want to be remembered for and what you are actually doing, that is a strong signal to treat your life purpose(s) with more respect. This is not an easy exercise, for it forces us to face our mortality, but I haven't met anyone who doesn't find it a strong motivator.

☙ Self-Esteem

Make a written list of things you do well—as many as you can think of, but at least five—no matter how small or large. Keep reading the list over and over until you have memorized it, and add more items as you think of them.

Now make a list of five or more things you like about yourself.

Next, write a list of your positive attributes, of anything good anyone has ever said about you, and any positive adjectives you can think of that apply to you. Ask a friend or family member for help with the list (and help them with theirs!). Write these lists out in big letters, and look at them at least once a day.

Below are a small handful of Dr. Nathaniel Branden's sentence-completion exercises. His books contain many more. For each sentence stem, write down six to ten completing phrases, without stopping to criticize or think about them. Then go over them and see what they mean to you. Warning: These can set off some powerful emotions.

If no one can give me good self-esteem except myself,

_____.

One of the things I can do to raise my self-esteem is

_____.

As I learn to accept myself,

_____.

One of the things I need to learn to accept is

_____.

I am becoming aware

_____.

If I take full responsibility for my actions,

_____.

If I take full responsibility for the things I say,

_____.

If I persist in blaming other people,

_____.

(Sources: Brandon, N. *Six Pillars of Self-Esteem*. New York: Bantam, 1994.
Brandon, N. *How to Raise Your Self-Esteem*. New York: Bantam, 1987.)

❧ Survival in the Hospital

(Adapted from Dr. Bernie Siegel's "Instructions for Hospitalized Patients"
in *Love, Medicine and Miracles*. New York: Harper & Row, 1986.)

Take comfortable clothes and wear them, instead of hospital gowns, when practical (to maintain your individuality).

Get a private room if you can afford it.

Don't get a room right next to the nurses' station (too noisy, unless you're in critical condition) or too far away (they might forget you).

Have family bring food from home, if it meets dietary requirements, unless you really like hospital food.

Have someone stay with you as much as possible, twenty-four hours a day if possible. (Make sure they know how to be quiet and are unafraid to question authority about tests and treatments.)

Walk as much as possible.

Take room decorations (personal and inspirational) with you.

Make sure your room has a window with a view.

Bring a tape recorder with music, relaxation tapes, and blank tapes for taping conversations with doctors.

If you undergo surgery, tell surgeons and anesthesiologists to repeat positive messages and avoid negative ones while you are in the operating room.

Get moving again as soon after surgery as you can. Walk; leave the hospital for outings.

❧ Generic Adaptation Strategy

This section gives a basic strategy for addressing functional problems associated with illness. I will use the issue of bladder control as an example, since so many people, including me, have problems with it. This discussion will focus on the principles involved, rather than specific techniques.

First, learn about the problem. Bladder problems can originate with neurological illness, muscle or nerve injury (often from childbirth), urological problems such as kidney stones, or the effects of medications. Apply appropriate self-care methods: Exercises can help strengthen sphincter control to avoid accidents; self-monitoring can show us what foods or drinks make the bladder twitchier, so we can avoid them. Since stress aggravates bladder spasms, we can use a relaxation program. We can ask our doctor for medicines that help reduce spasms or schedule our diuretics (water pills) for the most convenient times. We can look into herbs that have soothing effects on the bladder.

We can modify behavior to avoid accidents, for example, by making sure we use the bathroom any time we are about to leave a building and by planning routes with bathrooms nearby when we are out. Note: Don't cut down on liquids to avoid having to urinate. Dehydrating just makes the urine more concentrated and irritating to the bladder, while putting extra strain on the kidneys.

If necessary, we can wear absorbent undergarments, such as Depends. Staying home because we are unwilling to wear undergarments is like not going out because we don't want to be seen with a cane—this might be even more self-defeating, because nobody even sees our underwear!

We can use similar self-care principles to deal with other issues, including sleep, pain, mobility, bowel function, and eating difficulties. We can learn by reading books and asking our support groups. We can monitor ourselves, relax and reduce stress, or get some exercise if appropriate. We can ask for assistance from doctors, physical therapists, friends, or whoever can help; we can look into specialty equipment by checking out disability magazines and websites. We can research any medical or alternative therapies that claim to help our particular problem. We can modify behavior to help maintain function (e.g., eating smaller, more frequent meals if we can't tolerate large ones). Here's the key: We should be creative and refuse to give up.

⟿ *Medications* ⟾

In Healthier Living classes, when we ask participants what it is about their condition that most frustrates them, many answer, "The medications." Between side effects, ineffectiveness, expense, and the difficulty of actually keeping up with and taking them, medications often become a central focus of our lives, and that is no fun. Some doctors, especially cardiologists, prescribe ten or twelve different medications, which is usually excessive. Some people have multiple doctors, all prescribing different drugs. No doctor in the world could sort out the interactions between so many drugs, and precious few patients can keep them straight and take them correctly.

We should discuss medication problems with our doctors, keep a written list of meds with us, and make sure all our doctors and other practitioners know what meds we are on. To keep them straight, get a weekly pill dispenser from the pharmacy and fill it—or get someone else to fill it—at the beginning of each week. Connect taking medicines to a regular activity you do every day, like eating or watching the six-o'clock news.

If cost is a problem, ask your doctor if there is something cheaper that will work. Make sure you're getting generics, if they're available. Since larger doses usually cost only a little more than smaller ones, have the doc order larger pills that you can cut in half to get the correct dose.

Keep track of anything that occurs that you think might be a side effect, including the time this reaction comes on in relation to your medicine dose. Write these reactions down and discuss them with the doctor. Some medicines are worth the side effects, but we can do without some others or substitute for them. Please tell your doctor if you stop or change your meds; otherwise, he or she will have no clue what's going on and may order the wrong thing.

REFERENCES

⌒Chapter 1

⁓Not Our Fault⁓

Brauer, W., S. Merkesdal, and W. Mau. "Association of Disease Severity in the Early Course of Rheumatoid Arthritis and Locus of Control." *Psychother Psychosom Med Psychol*, 51(8) (2001): 320–7.

Buckelew, S.P., B. Huyser, et al. "Self-efficacy Predicting Outcome Among Fibromyalgia Subjects." *Arthritis Care Res*, 9 (1996): 97–104.

Burckhardt, C.S. "The Impact of Arthritis on Quality of Life." *Nurs Res*, 34 (1985): 11–16.

Chen, C.C., A.S. David, H. Nunnerley, M. Michell, J.L. Dawson, H. Berry, J. Dobbs, and T. Fahy. "Adverse Life Events and Cancer." *British Medical Journal*, 311 (1995): 1527–1530.

Coughlin, A.M., A.S. Badura, T.D. Fleischer, and T.P. Guck. "Multidisciplinary Treatment of Chronic Pain Patients: Its Efficacy in Changing Patient Locus of Control." *Arch Phys Med Rehabil*, 81 (2000): 739–740.

DeLongis, A., et al. "Relationship of Daily Hassles, Uplifts, and Major Life Events to Health Status." *Health Psychology*, 1 (1982): 119.

Van den Akker, M., F. Buntinx, J.F. Metsemakers, and J.A. Knottnerus. "Psychosocial Patient Characteristics and GP-registered Chronic Morbidity: A Prospective Study." *J Psychosom Res*, 50 (2001): 95–102.

⁓Health Reflects Life⁓

Adler, N.E., T. Boyce, M.A. Chesney, S. Cohen, S. Folkman, R.L. Kahn, and S.L. Syme. "Socioeconomic Status and Health: The Challenge of the Gradient." *American Psychologist*, 49 (1994): 15–24.

Bartrop, R.W., E. Luckhurst, L. Lazarus, L.G. Kiloh, and R. Penny. "Depressed Lymphocyte Function After Bereavement." *Lancet* 1 (8016) (1977): 834–836.

Cohen, S. et al. "Psychological Stress and Susceptibility to the Common Cold." *New England J of Medicine*, 325 (1991): 606–612.

Coyne J.C., M.J. Rohrbaugh, et al. "Prognostic Importance of Marital Quality for Survival of Congestive Heart Failure." *Am J Cardiol*, 88 (2001): 526–529.

Lebowitz, M. "The Relationship of Socio-environmental Factors to the Prevalence of Obstructive Lung Diseases and Other Chronic Conditions." *J of Chronic Diseases*, 30 (1977): 599–611.

Lynch, J., G. Kaplan, and S. Shema. "Cumulative Impact of Sustained Economic Hardship on Physical, Cognitive, Psychological and Social Functioning." *New England J of Medicine*, 337 (1997): 1889–1895.

Nortveldt, M.W., T. Riise, J. M. Myhr, and H.I. Nyland. "Quality of Life as a Predictor for Change in Disability in MS." *Neurology*, 55 (2000): 51–54.

Ornstein, Robert and David Sobel. *Healthy Pleasures*. Reading, MA: Addison-Wesley, 1987, pp. 76–78.

Schwartz, G.E. and L.G. Russek. "Perceptions of Parental Caring Predict Health Status in Midlife: A 35-Year Follow-Up Study of the Harvard Stress Study." *Psychosomatic Medicine*, 59 (1997): 144–149.

Tan, S.A., L.G. Tan, L.S. Berk, S.T. Lukman, and L.F. Lukman. "Mirthful Laughter: An Effective Adjunct in Cardiac Rehabilitation." *Canadian J of Cardiology*, 13 (Supp B) (1997): 190B.

⌒ *My Ticket Out of Here* ⌒

Patton, R., and L. Gardner. "Influence of Family Environment on Growth: The Syndrome of Maternal Deprivation." *Pediatrics*, 30 (1962): 957–962.

⌒ *The Activity/Pain Cycle* ⌒

Keefe, F., P. Beaupre, and K. Gil. "Group Therapy for Patients with Chronic Pain." In *Psychological Approaches to Pain Management, A Practitioner's Handbook*. R. Gatchel and D. Turk (eds.). New York: Guilford (1997): 272–274.

⌒ *Cost/Benefit Analysis* ⌒

Haan, M., G.A. Kaplan, and T. Camacho. "Poverty and Health: Prospective Evidence from the Alameda County Study." *Am J of Epidemiology*, 125 (1987): 989–998.

Myers, A.H., B. Rosner, H. Abbey, W. Willet, M.J. Stampfer, C. Bain, R. Lipnick, C. Hennekens, and F. Speizer. "Smoking Behavior Among Participants in the Nurses' Health Study." *Am J of Public Health,* 77 (1987): 628–630.

Pincus, T., R. Esther, D. DeWalt, and L. Callahan. "Social Conditions and Self-Management Are More Powerful Determinants of Health Than Access to Care." *Annals of Internal Medicine,* 129 (1998): 406–411.

⟶ *Barriers to Self-Care* ⟶

Feste, Catherine. *The Physician Within (2nd ed.).* New York: Henry Holt, 1993, pp. 19–44.

⟶ *Loss of Hope* ⟶

Everson, S.A., G.A. Kaplan, D.E. Goldbert, and J.T. Salonen. "Hypertension Incidence Is Predicted by High Levels of Hopelessness in Finnish Men." *Hypertension,* 35 (2000): 561–567.

Lewis, S.C., M.S. Dennis, S.J. O'Rourke, and M. Sharpe. "Negative Attitudes Among Short-term Stroke Survivors Predict Worse Long-term Survival." *Stroke,* 32 (2001): 1640–1645.

Feste, pp. 56–61.

Siegel, Bernie. *Love, Medicine and Miracles.* New York: Harper & Row, 1986, pp. 36–43.

⟶ *The Riddle of Compliance* ⟶

Feste, p. 150.

Horwitz, R.I., and S.M. Horwitz. "Adherence to Treatment and Health Outcomes." *Archives of Internal Medicine,* 153 (1993): 1863–1868.

Volmink, J., and P. Garner. "Systematic Review of Randomized Controlled Trials of Strategies to Promote Adherence to Tuberculosis Treatment." *BMJ,* 315 (7120) (1997): 1403–1406.

⟶ *Why We Need Doctors* ⟶

Babyak, M., J.A. Blumenthal, et al. "Exercise Treatment for Major Depression: Maintenance of Therapeutic Benefit at 10 Months." *Psychosom Med,* 62 (2000): 633–638.

Ornish, D.M. et al "Can Lifestyle Change Reverse Coronary Heart Disease? The Lifestyle Heart Trial," *Lancet*, 336 (1990): 129–133.

Singh, N.A., K.M. Clements, and M.A. Singh. "The Efficacy of Exercise as a Long-term Antidepressant in Elderly Subjects: A Randomized, Controlled Trial." *J Gerontol A Biol Sci Med Sci*, 56 (2001): M497–504.

☞ *Recovery Yes; Cure Maybe* ☜

Lorig, K., D. Lubeck, R.G. Kraines, M. Seleznick, and H.R. Holman. "Outcomes of Self-help Education for Patients with Arthritis." *Arthritis and Rheumatism*, 28 (1985): 680–685.

Lorig, K., D. Sobel, et al. "Evidence Suggesting that a Chronic Disease Self-management Program Can Improve Health Status while Reducing Hospitalization: A Randomized Trial." *Medical Care*, 37 (1999): 5–14.

Salaffi, F., F. Cavalieri, M. Nolli, and G. Ferraccioli. "Analysis of Disability in Known Osteoarthritis: Relationship with Age and Psychological Variables but Not with Radiographic Score." *Journal of Rheumatology*, 18 (1991): 1581–1586.

☞ Chapter 2

☞ *"I Don't Have Time, I Don't Have Time"* ☜

Crowther, J.H. "Stress Management Training and Relaxation Imagery in the Treatment of Essential Hypertension." *J of Behavioral Med*, 6 (1983): 169–187.

Hyman, R.B., H.R. Feldman, R.B. Harris, R.F. Levin, and G.B. Malloy. "Effect of Relaxation Training on Clinical Symptoms: A Meta-analysis." *Nursing Research*, 38 (1989): 216–220.

Martin, P. *The Healing Mind*. New York: St. Martin's Press, 1997, pp. 19–26.

Sharpe, M. "Cognitive Behavior Therapy for Chronic Fatigue." *British Medical Journal*, 312 (1996): 22–26.

☞ *Time's Bullet Train* ☜

Whitrow, G.J. *What Is Time?* London: Thames and Hudson, 1972, pp. 7–25.

⟶ *Living on the Dog Track* ⟵

Martin, P., pp. 19–26.

Sapolsky, R.M. *Why Zebras Don't Get Ulcers: A Guide to Stress, Stress-Related Diseases, and Coping.* New York: Macmillan, 1994, pp. 31–36.

⟶ *What's Wrong with Stress?* ⟵

Bennett E.J., C.C. Tennant, C. Piesse, C.A. Badcock, and J.E. Kellow. "Level of Chronic Life Stress Predicts Clinical Outcome in Irritable Bowel Syndrome." *Gut,* 43 (1998): 256–261.

Herrmann, M., J. Scholmerich, and R.H. Straub. "Stress and Rheumatic Diseases." *Rheum Dis Clin North Am,* 26 (2000): 737–763.

Jiang, W., et al. "Mental Stress-Induced Myocardial Ischemia and Cardiac Events." *J Am Medical Association,* 175 (1996): 1651–1656.

Kiecolt-Glazer, et al. "Spousal Caregivers of Dementia Victims—Changes in Immunity and Health." *Psychosomatic Medicine,* 53 (1991): 345–362.

Marucha, P.T., J.K. Kiecolt-Glaser, and M. Favagehi. "Mucosal Wound Healing is Impaired by Examination Stress." *Psychosomatic Medicine,* 60 (1998): 362–365.

Mohr, D.C., D.E. Goodkin, et al. "Psychological Stress and the Subsequent Appearance of New Brain MRI Lesions in MS." *Neurology,* 55 (2000): 55–61.

Rich-Edwards, J., N. Krieger, J. Majzoub, S. Zierler, E. Lieberman, and M. Gillman. "Maternal Experiences of Racism and Violence as Predictors of Preterm Birth: Rationale and Study Design." *Paediatr Perinat Epidemiol,* 15 Suppl 2 (2001): 124–135.

⟶ *Conscious Breathing* ⟵

Benson, Herbert. *The Relaxation Response.* New York: Morrow, 1975.

Goodale I.L., A.D. Domar, and H. Benson. "Alleviation of Premenstrual Syndrome Symptoms with the Relaxation Response." *Obstetrics and Gynecology,* 75 (1990): 649–655.

Kabat-Zinn, J., L. Lipworth, and R. Burney. "The Clinical Use of Mindfulness Meditation for the Self-regulation of Chronic Pain." *Journal of Behavioral Medicine,* 8 (1985): 163–190.

Keating, Fr. Thomas. *Open Mind, Open Heart.* London: Harper Collins UK, 1994.

Remember the Sabbath

Blumenthal, J., et al. "Stress Management and Exercise Training in Cardiac Patients with Myocardial Ischemia: Effects on Prognosis and Evaluation of Mechanisms." *Archives of Internal Medicine*, 157 (1997): 2213–2223.

Muller, W. *Sabbath: Restoring the Sacred Rhythm of Rest*. New York: Bantam Doubleday Dell, 1999.

Patel, C., and M. Marmot. "Stress Management, Blood Pressure and Quality of Life." *J of Hypertension*, 5 Supp 1 (1987): S21–S28.

Awareness Is Its Own Reward

Benson, H., pp. 119–120.

Kuralt, C. *On the Road*. New York: Putnam and Sons, 1985, p. 53.

Chapter 3

Any Change at All

Lorig, K., D. Lubeck, M. Seleznick, B.W. Brown Jr., E. Ung, and H.R. Holman. "The Beneficial Outcomes of the Arthritis Self-management Course Are Inadequately Explained by Behavior Change." *Arthritis and Rheumatism*, 31 (1989): 91–95.

O'Leary, A. "Self-efficacy and Health." *Behavioral Research and Therapy*, 23 (1985): 437–451.

How Change Works

Lorig, K., H. Halsted, D. Sobel, D. Laurent, V. Gonzalez, and M. Minor. *Living a Healthy Life with Chronic Conditions*. Palo Alto, CA: Bull Publishing, 1994, pp. 17–28.

Habit Control

Borland, R., C.J. Segan, P.M. Livingston, and N. Owen. "The Effectiveness of Callback Counseling for Smoking Cessation: A Randomized Trial." *Addiction*, 96 (6) (2001): 881–889.

Diamond, J. "Making Friends with Your Addiction." *Family Therapy Networker*, July/August 2000: 40–47.

Wadland, W.C., B. Soffelmayr, and K. Ives. "Enhancing Smoking Cessation of Low-income Smokers in Managed Care." *J Fam Pract*, 50 (2001): 138–144.

⟶ *Healthy and Unhealthy Beliefs* ⟵

Conner, M., and P. Norman. *Predicting Health Behaviours: Research and Practice with Social Cognition Models.* Buckingham, U.K.: Open University Press, 1995.

Radnitz, C. (ed.). *Cognitive-Behavioral Therapy for Persons with Disabilities.* Northvale, NJ: Jason Aronson, 2000.

Simonton, C., and S. Matthews-Simonton. "Belief Systems and Management of the Emotional Aspects of Malignancy." *Journal of Transpersonal Psychology,* 7 (1975): 29–47.

⟶ *Take This Job, Please* ⟵

Frymoyer, J., and W. Cats-Batil. "Identifying Patients at Risk for Becoming Disabled." *Spine*, 16 (1991): 605–607.

Frymoyer, J., and W. Cats-Batil. "Predictors of Low Back Pain Disability." *Clinical Orthopedics*, 221 (1987): 89–98.

Marmot, M.C. "Employment Grade and Coronary Heart Disease in Civil Servants." *Journal of Edpidemiology and Community Health*, 32 (1978): 244.

Marmot, M.G., H. Bosma, H. Hemingway, Brunner, and S. Stansfeld. "Contribution of Job Control and Other Risk Factors to Social Variations in Coronary Heart Disease Incidence." *The Lancet*, 350 (1997): 235–239.

Schernhammer, E.S., F. Laden, et al. "Rotating Night Shifts and Risk of Breast Cancer in Women Participating in the Nurses' Health Study." *J Natl Cancer Inst*, 93 (2001): 1563–1568.

⟶ *The Meaning of Our Work* ⟵

Feuerstein, M. "Workstyle: Definition, Empirical Support and Implications for Prevention, Evaluation, and Rehabilitation of Occupational Upper Extremity Disorders." In *Beyond Biomechanics: Psychosocial Aspects of Musculoskeletal Disorders in Office Work*, S. Moon and S. Sauter (eds.). (1996) 177–206.

Fitzgerald, T. "Pain-Related Occupational Musculoskeletal Disability." In *Cognitive-Behavioral Therapy for Persons with Disabilities*. C. Radnitz (ed.). Northvale, NJ: Jason Aronson, Inc., 2000, pp. 77–104.

✐ *Knowing When to Quit* ✐

Martikainen, P. "Unemployment and Mortality." *British Medical Journal,* 301 (1990): 407.

Wilson, S.H., and G.M. Walker. "Unemployment and Health." *Public Health,* 107 (1993): 153–162.

✐ *Relationships* ✐

Barasch, M.I., and C. Hershberg. *Remarkable Recovery.* New York: Riverhead Books, 1995, pp. 210–225.

Kiecolt-Glaser, J., et al. "Negative Behavior During Marital Conflict and Immunological Down-regulation." *Psychosomatic Medicine,* 55 (1993): 395–409.

Lynch, J. *A Cry Unheard: New Insights into the Medical Consequences of Loneliness.* Baltimore, MD: Bancroft, 2000.

Weiss, R.G., and B.M. Aved. "Marital Satisfaction and Depression as a Predictor of Physical Health." *Journal of Consulting Clinical Psychiatry,* 46 (1978): 1379.

✐ *Places of Refuge* ✐

Kellett, J. "Health and Housing." *J of Psychosomatic Research,* 33 (1989): 255–268.

Thomson, H., M. Petticrew, and D. Morrison. "Health Effects of Housing Improvement: Systematic Review of Intervention Studies." *BMJ,* 323 (2001): 187–190.

✐ Chapter 4

✐ *All the Help We Can Get* ✐

Berkman, L.F., and S.L. Syme. "Social Networks, Host Resistance, and Mortality: A Nine-year Followup Study of Alameda County Residents." *American J of Epidemiology,* 109 (1979): 186–204.

Maunsell, E., et al. "Social Support and Survival Among Women with Breast Cancer." *Cancer,* 76 (1995): 631–637.

Orth-Gomer, K., and J. Johnson. "Social Network Interaction and Mortality," *J of Chronic Diseases,* 40 (1987): 949–957.

Orth-Gomer, K., A. Rosengren, and L. Wilhelmsen. "Lack of Social Support and Incidence of Coronary Heart Disease in Middle-aged Swedish Men." *Psychosomatic Medicine*, 55 (1993): 37–43.

The John Wayne Syndrome

Register, C. *The Chronic Illness Experience: Embracing the Imperfect Life.* Center City, MN: Hazelden, 1999, pp. 63–74.

Religious and Voluntary Organizations

Byrd, R.C. "Positive Therapeutic Effects of Intercessory Prayer in a Coronary Care Unit Population." *Southern Medical J*, 81 (1988): 826–829.

Cha, K.Y., D.P Wirth, and R.A. Lobo. "Does Prayer Influence the Success of in Vitro Fertilization—Embryo Transfer? Report of a Masked, Randomized Trial." *J Reprod Med*, 46 (2001): 781–787.

Sicher, F., E. Targ, D. Moore II, and H.S. Smith. "A Randomized Double-blind Study of the Effect of Distant Healing in a Population with Advanced AIDS." *Western J of Medicine*, 169 (1998): 356–363.

Support Groups

Fawzy, F., et al. "Malignant Melanoma: Effects of an Early Structured Psychiatric Intervention, Coping and Affective State on Recurrence and Survival 6 Years Later." *Archives of General Psychiatry*, 50 (1993): 681–689.

Fawzy, F., et al. "Psychosocial Interventions in Cancer Care." *Archives of General Psychiatry*, 52 (1995): 100–113.

Spiegel, D., J. Bloom, et al. "Effects of Psychosocial Treatment on Survival of Patients with Metastatic Breast Cancer." *Lancet*, 2 (1989): 888–891.

Health Professionals

Armstrong, L., with S. Jenkins. *It's Not About the Bike.* New York: G.P. Putnam, 2000, pp. 101–104.

Siegel, B. *Love, Medicine and Miracles.* New York: Harper & Row, 1986, pp. 27–28.

↶ *Get the Most from Your Healers* ↶

Kohn, L., M. Donaldson, and J. Corrigan (eds.). "To Err is Human." Institute of Medicine Report, 1999.

↶ *Assertiveness* ↶

Albert Ellis, quoted in Spero, A.J., and B. Wittman. *The Project Eve Leaders' Guidebook*. Buffalo: University of the State of New York, 1981, p. 33.
Richardson, C. *Take Time for Your Life*. New York: Broadway Books, 1998, p. 73.

↶ *Disclosure* ↶

Goleman, D. *Emotional Intelligence*. New York: Bantam Books, 1995.

↶ *How to Ask for Help* ↶

Lorig, K., H. Halsted, D. Sobel, D. Laurent, V. Gonzalez, and M. Minor. *Living a Healthy Life with Chronic Conditions*. Palo Alto, CA: Bull Publishing, 1994, p. 133.

↶ Chapter 5

↶ *Twenty-Four Reasons to Live* ↶

Langer, E., and D. Rodin. "The Effects of Choice and Enhanced Personal Responsibility for the Aged: A Field Experiment in an Institutional Setting." *J of Personality and Social Psychology*, 34 (1976): 191–198.
Langer, E., and D. Rodin. "Long Term Effect of a Control-relevant Intervention with the Institutionalized Aged." *J of Personality and Social Psychology*, 35 (1977): 897–902.
Stones, M.J., B. Dornan, and A. Kozma. "The Prediction of Mortality in Elderly Institution Residents." *J Gerontol*, 44 (3) (1989): 72–79.

↶ *I'm Focused; You're Obsessed* ↶

Llamas, M.V. *Claudia*. Morales Mexico DF: Plaza & Janés Editores, 1998.

⟿ *Work Necessary, Job Optional* ⟿

LeShan, L. *Cancer as a Turning Point*. New York: Dutton, 1989.

Thoits, P.A., and L.N. Hewitt. "Volunteer Work and Well-being." *J Health Soc Behav*, 42 (2001): 115–131.

⟿ *Faith and Spirit* ⟿

Levin, et al. "Religious Effects on Health Status Among Black Americans." *J Gerontol B Psychol Sci Soc Sci.*, 50 (1995): S154–163.

McCullough, M., et al. "Religious Involvement and Mortality: A Meta-Analytic Review." *Health Psychology*, 19 (2000): 211–222.

Payne, I., A. Bergin, K. Belema, and P. Jenksin. "Review of Religion and Mental Health." *Prevention in Human Services*, 9 (1991): 11–40.

Simonton, C., and S. Matthews-Simonton. "Belief Systems and Management of the Emotional Aspects of Malignancy." *J of Transpersonal Psychology*, 7 (1975): 29–47.

⟿ *What About Love?* ⟿

Kravdal, O. "The Impact of Marital Status on Cancer Survival." *Soc Sci Med*, 52 (2001): 357–368.

Sobel, D. "Rx Love." *Mind/Body Health Newsletter*, 9 (2) (2000): 1.

⟿ *Love and Sex* ⟿

Davey Smith, G., S. Frankel, and J. Yarnell. "Sex and Death: Are They Related? Findings from the Caerphilly Cohort Study." *British Medical Journal*, 315 (7123) (1997): 1641–1644.

Muller, J.E., M.A. Mittleman, et al. "Triggering Myocardial Infarction by Sexual Activity: Low Absolute Risk and Prevention by Regular Physical Exertion?" *J of the Am Medical Association*, 275 (1996): 1405–1409.

Sachs, J. *The Healing Power of Sex*. Des Moines, IA: Prentice-Hall, 1994, p. 17.

⟿ *Keep Looking Ahead* ⟿

Martin, P. *The Healing Mind*. New York: St. Martin's Press, 1997, p. 6.

Phillips, D.P., and D.G. Smith. "Postponement of Death Until Symbolically Meaningful Occasions." *J of Am Medical Association*, 163 (1990): 1947–1951.

❧ *Pleasure Is Good for You* ❧

Doll, R. "One for the Heart." *British Medical Journal*, 315 (1997): 1664–1668.

Koivumaa-Honkanen, H., R. Honkanen, H. Viinamaki, K. Heikkila, J. Kaprio, and M. Koskenvuo. "Self-reported Life Satisfaction and 20-year Mortality in Healthy Finnish Adults." *Am J Epidemiol*, 152 (2000): 983–991.

Lee, I.M., and R.S. Paffenbarger. "Life is Sweet: Candy Consumption and Longevity." *British Medical Journal*, 317 (1998): 1683–1684.

Ornstein, R., and D. Sobel. *Healthy Pleasures.* Reading, MA: Addison-Wesley, 1987.

Waterhouse, A.L., et al. "Antioxidants in Chocolate," *Lancet*, 348 (9030) (1996): 834.

❧ *Fun Therapy* ❧

Cousins, N. *Anatomy of an Illness as Perceived by the Patient.* New York: W.W. Norton, 1979.

Tan, S.A., L.G. Tan, et al. "Mirthful Laughter: An Effective Adjunct in Cardiac Rehabilitation." *Canadian J of Cardiology*, 13 Supp B (1997): 190B.

❧ *The Incredible Power of Pets* ❧

Allen, K.M., et al. "Presence of Human Friends and Pet Dogs as Moderators of Autonomic Response to Stress in Women." *J of Personality and Social Psychology*, 61(1991): 582–589.

Friedmann, E., A. Katcher, J.J. Lynch, and S.A. Thomas. "Animal Companions and One-year Survival of Patients After Discharge from a Coronary Care Unit." *Public Health Reports*, 95: 307–312 (1980).

Friedmann, E., and S.A. Thomas. "Pet Ownership, Social Support, and One-year Survival After Acute Myocardial Infarction in the Cardiac Arrhythmia Suppression Trial (CAST)." *Am J Cardiology*, 76 (1995): 1213–1217.

❧ *Siesta Time* ❧

Trichopoulos, D., A. Tzonou, et al. "Does a Siesta Protect from Coronary Heart Disease?" *Lancet*, Aug 1; 2 (1987): 269–270.

⟶ *Go See Your Mother* ⟶

Nagpal, S., J. Lu, and M.F. Boehm. "Vitamin D Analogs: Mechanism of Action and Therapeutic Applications." *Curr Med Chem*, (2001): 1679–1697.

⟶ *Back to School* ⟶

Mulcahy, R., L. Daley, et al. "Level of Education, Coronary Risk Factors, and Cardiovascular Disease." *Irish Medical Journal*, 77 (1984): 316–318.

Ornstein, R., and D. Sobel, pp. 190–194.

Pincus, T., L. Callahan, and R. Burkhauser. "Most Chronic Diseases are Reported More Frequently in Individuals with Fewer than 12 Years of Formal Education in the 18–64 United States Population." *J of Chronic Diseases*, 40 (1987): 865–874.

White, L., R. Katzman, et al. "Association of Education with Incidence of Cognitive Impairment in Three Established Populations for Epidemiologic Studies of the Elderly." *J of Clinical Epidemiology*, 47 (1994): 363–374.

⟶ Chapter 6

⟶ *Growing Up Under Fire* ⟶

Greer, S., T. Morris, and K.W. Pettingale. "Psychological Response to Breast Cancer: Effect on Outcome." *Lancet*, 2 (8146) (1979): 785–787.

Siegel, B., pp. 51–54.

Tschuschke, V., B. Hertenstein, et al. "Associations Between Coping and Survival Time of Adult Leukemia Patients Receiving Allogeneic Bone Marrow Transplantation: Results." *J Psychosomatic Research*, 50 (5) (2001): 277–285.

⟶ *The Myth of the Exceptional Patient* ⟶

Siegel, B., pp. 22–26.

⟶ *More Control Than We Think* ⟶

Cousins, N. *The Healing Heart*. New York: W.W. Norton, 1983.

Greenfield, S., S. Kaplan, and J.E. Ware. "Expanding Patient Involvement in Care: Effects on Patient Outcomes." *Annals of Internal Medicine*, 102 (1985): 520–528.

Holden-Lund, C. "Effects of Relaxation with Guided Imagery on Surgical Stress and Wound Healing." *Research in Nursing and Health*, 11 (1988): 235–244.

Kuhn, B.R., M.D. Shriver, and K.D. Allen. "Behavioral Management of Children's Seizure Activity: Intervention Guidelines for Primary-care Providers." *Clinical Pediatrics*, 34 (1995): 570–575.

Ornish, D.M. et al "Can Lifestyle Change Reverse Coronary Heart Disease? The Lifestyle Heart Trial." *Lancet*, 336 (1990): 129–133.

Vickery, D.M., H. Kalmer, D. Lowry, et al: "Effect of a Self-care Education Program on Medical Visits." *J Am Medical Association*, 250 (1983): 2952–2956.

Wauquier, A., A. McGrady, et al. "Changes in Cerebral Blood Flow Velocity Associated with Biofeedback-assisted Relaxation Treatment of Migraine Headaches are Specific for the Middle Cerebral Artery." *Headache*, 35 (1995): 358–362.

⌒ *How Much Responsibility Can I Take?* ⌒

Linton, S.J., and T. Andersson. "Can Chronic Disability be Prevented? A Randomized Trial of Cognitive-behavior Intervention and Two Forms of Information for Patients with Spinal Pain." *Spine*, 25 (2000): 2825–2831.

Richard, A. "Self-Help for Seizures." *Medical Self-Care*, May/June 1988. 45–51.

⌒ *Arm Yourself with Knowledge* ⌒

Royer, A. *Life with Chronic Illness: Social and Psychological Dimensions*. St. Louis: Praeger, 1998, p. 92.

⌒ *How Much Am I Worth?* ⌒

Branden, N. *Six Pillars of Self-Esteem*. New York: Bantam, 1994, pp. 3–25.

⌒ *Forgiveness Begins at Home* ⌒

Festa, L.M., and I. Tuck. "A Review of Forgiveness Literature with Implications for Nursing Practice." *Holistic Nursing Practice*, 14 (4) (2000): 77–86.

⟋ *If You Were a Stock, I'd Buy Two Hundred Shares* ⟍

Branden, N. *How to Raise Your Self-Esteem.* New York: Bantam, 1987.

⟋ *Stages of Acceptance* ⟍

Register, C. *The Chronic Illness Experience: Embracing the Imperfect Life.* Center City, MN: Hazelden, 1999, p. 23.

⟋ Chapter 7

⟋ *Your Body—Love It or Leave It* ⟍

McCrum, Robert. *My Year Off.* New York: W.W. Norton, 1998, p. 50.

⟋ *The Body Remembers* ⟍

Bunzel, B., et al "Does Changing the Heart Mean Changing Personality? A Retrospective Inquiry on 47 Heart Transplant Patients." *Quality of Life Research,* 1 (1992): 251–256.

Johnson, D. *The Protean Body.* New York: Harper Colophon, 1977, pp. 26–29.

⟋ *Where Does Emotion Come From?* ⟍

Atkinson, B. "The Emotional Imperative." *Family Therapy Networker,* July/Aug 1999: 22–33.

Pert, C. *Molecules of Emotion.* New York: Simon and Schuster, 1999, pp. 130–149.

Pert, C.B., et al. "Neuropeptides and Their Receptors: A Psychosomatic Network," *Journal of Immunology,* 135 (1985): 820S–826S.

Shapiro, D. *Your Body Speaks Your Mind.* Santa Cruz, CA: Crossing Press. 1997.

⟋ *The Body Wakes Us Up* ⟍

McCrum, R., p. 172.

Obelieniene, D., H. Schrader, et al. "Pain after Whiplash: a Prospective Controlled Inception Cohort Study." *Journal of Neurology, Neurosurgery and Psychiatry* 66 (1999): 279–283.

Rainville, J., J.B. Sobel, C. Hartigan, and A. Wright. "The Effect of Compensation Involvement on the Reporting of Pain and Disability by Patients Referred for Rehabilitation of Chronic Low Back Pain." *Spine,* 22 (1997): 2016–2024.

── *The Incredible Immune System* ──

Martin, P., pp. 65–80.

── *The Body Goes Food Shopping* ──

Kleinman, R. *Let Them Eat Cake: The Case Against Controlling What Your Children Eat.* New York: Villard, 1994.

Roth, G. *Breaking Free from Compulsive Eating.* New York: Plume, 1993.

Roth, G. *When Food Is Love.* New York: Plume, 1993.

── *What Does Illness Want?* ──

Rossman, M. *Guided Imagery for Self-Healing.* Novato, CA: New World Library, 2000, pp. 115–116.

Shapiro, D. *Your Body Speaks Your Mind.* Santa Cruz, CA: Crossing Press, 1997.

── *Imagery: Language of the Body* ──

Barasch, M.I. *Healing Dreams.* New York: Riverhead Press, 2000, pp. 1–5.

── *Who's Driving the Car?* ──

Assagioli, R. *Psychosynthesis.* New York: Hobbs Dorman, 1965.

Evans, C., and P.H. Richardson. "Improved Recovery and Reduced Postoperative Stay After Therapeutic Suggestions During General Anesthesia." *Lancet,* 2 (8609) (1988): 491–493.

McLintock, T.T., et al "Postoperative Analgesic Requirements in Patients Exposed to Positive Intraoperative Suggestions." *BMJ,* 301 (1990) 788–790.

Siegel, B., pp. 45–51.

⚬ *Pain: The Mind/Body's Tightest Link* ⚬

Bresler, D. *Free Yourself from Pain.* New York: Simon and Schuster, 1979.

Cohen, D. *Arthritis, Stop Suffering, Start Moving.* New York: Walker and Company, 1995.

Materson, R. "The Stress-Pain Relationship." *The Pain Practitioner,* 9 (4) (1999): 1–3.

Reid, G.J., and P.J. McGrath. "Psychological Treatments for Migraine." *Biomed Pharmacothera,* 50 (1996): 58–63.

Syrjala, K.L., G.W. Donaldson, M.W. Davis, M.E. Kippes, and J.E. Carr. "Relaxation and Imagery and Cognitive-behavioral Training Reduce Pain During Cancer Treatment: A Controlled Clinical Trial." *Pain,* 63 (1995): 189–198.

⚬ *Emotional and Physical Pain* ⚬

Sarno, J. *The Mindbody Prescription.* New York: Warner Books, 1998.

⚬ *The Zen Master's Knees* ⚬

Shapiro, D., pp. 96–99.

⚬ Chapter 8

⚬ *Anger, Acceptance, Denial, Grief...* ⚬

Goleman, D. "Positive Denial: The Case for Not Facing Reality." *Psychology Today,* 13 (1979): 44–60.

Kübler-Ross, E. *On Death and Dying.* New York: Macmillan, 1969.

⚬ *Anger for Good and Ill* ⚬

Cohen, D. *Finding A Joyful Life in the Heart of Pain.* Boston, MA: Shambhala, 2000.

⟶ *Rhythm Is Life* ⟵

Mohr, D.C., D.E. Goodkin, et al. "Psychological Stress and the Subsequent Appearance of New Brain MRI Lesions in MS." *Neurology*, 55–61 (2000).

⟶ *Power of the Drum* ⟵

Barasch, M., and C. Hirschberg. *Remarkable Recovery*. New York: Riverhead Books, 1995, pp. 268–269.

Bernstein, B., and G. Johnson. "Rhythm Playing Characteristics in Persons with Severe Dementia Including Those with Probably Alzheimer's Type." *Journal of Music Therapy*, 1995: 113–131.

Friedman, R.L. *The Healing Power of the Drum*. Reno, NV: White Cliffs Media, 2000, pp. 62–63.

⟶ *Able-Heartedness* ⟵

Lemaistre, J. *Beyond Rage*. Oak Park, IL: Alpine Guild, 1985, p. 25.

⟶ *"We're Dancing Inside Our Shells"* ⟵

Stevenson, J. *Clams Can't Sing*. New York: Greenwillow Books, 1980.

☙ Chapter 9

⟶ *Get Moving* ⟵

Salmon, P. "Effects of Physical Exercise on Anxiety, Depression, and Sensitivity to Stress: A Unifying Theory." *Clin Psychol Rev*, 21 (2001): 33–61.

⟶ *Yoga* ⟵

Garfinkel, M.S., H.R. Schumacher Jr, A. Husain, et al. "Evaluation of a Yoga-based Regimen for Treatment of Osteoarthritis of the Hands." *J Rheumatol*, 21 (1994): 2341–2343.

⚊ *The Benefits of Strength* ⚊

Singh, N.A., K.M. Clements, and M.A. Fiatarone. "A Randomized Controlled Trial of Progressive Resistance Training in Depressed Elders." *J Gerontol A Biol Sci Med Sci*, 52 (1997): M27–35.

⚊ *Mental Self-Care* ⚊

Ikemi, Y., and S. Nakagawa. "A Psychosomatic Study of Contagious Dermatitis." *Kyoshu Journal of Medical Science*, 13 (1962): 335–350.

⚊ *Expression of Feelings* ⚊

Pennebaker, et al. "Disclosure of Traumas and Immune Function." *J of Consulting Clinical Psychiatry*, 56(1988): 239.

Smyth, J.M., A.A. Stone, A. Hurewitz, and A. Kaell. "Effects of Writing about Stressful Experiences on Symptom Reduction in Patients with Asthma and Rheumatoid Arthritis." *J of the American Medical Association*, 281 (1999): 1304–09.

⚊ *Mental Exercise* ⚊

Butler, S.M., J.W. Ashford, and D.A. Snowdon. "Age, Education, and Changes in the Mini-Mental State Exam Scores of Older Women: Findings from the Nun Study." *J Am Geriatr Soc*, 44 (1996): 675–681.

⚊ *Conscious Eating, Not Dieting* ⚊

Lorig, K., H. Halsted, D. Sobel, D. Laurent, V. Gonzalez, and M. Minor. *Living a Healthy Life with Chronic Conditions*. Palo Alto, CA: Bull Publishing, 1994, pp. 153–168.

Mellin, L. *The Solution*. New York: Harper Collins, 1997, pp. 1–30.

Roth, G. *Breaking Free from Compulsive Eating*. New York: Plume, 1993.

☙Chapter 10

⚬ *Evaluating Potential Treatments* ⚬

Lorig, K., V. Gonzalez, and D. Laurent. Stanford Patient Education Center, *The Healthy Living with Chronic Conditions Leaders' Guide*. Palo Alto, CA: Stanford University, 1999.

⚬ *Placebo Power* ⚬

Brody, H., and D Brody. *The Placebo Response: How You Can Release the Body's Inner Pharmacy for Better Health*. New York: Cliff Street Books, 2000.

⚬ *Bodywork* ⚬

Field, T. "Massage Therapy Effects." *American Psychologist*, 53 (1998): 1270–1281.

⚬ *Acupuncture* ⚬

Lu, D.P., G.P. Lu, and L. Kleinman. "Acupuncture and Clinical Hypnosis for Facial and Head and Neck Pain: A Single Crossover Comparison." *Am J Clin Hypn*, 44 (2001): 141–148.

⚬ *Reiki and Energy Work* ⚬

Sneed, N.V., M. Olson, B. Bubolz, and N. Finch. "Influences of a Relaxation Intervention on Perceived Stress and Power Spectral Analysis of Heart Rate Variability." *Prog Cardiovasc Nurs*, 16 (2001): 57–64, 79.

⚬ *Faith Healing and Shamans* ⚬

Bandura, A. *Self-Efficacy: The Exercise of Control*. New York: W.H. Freeman, 1997.

Branden, N. *Six Pillars of Self-Esteem*. New York: Bantam, 1994.

Branden, N. *How to Raise Your Self-Esteem*. New York: Bantam, 1987.

Friedman, M., and D. Ulmer. *Treating Type A Behavior—and Your Heart*. New York: Knopf, 1984.

Kirkpatrick, R.A. "Witchcraft and Lupus Erythematosus." *J of the American Medical Association*, 245 (1981): 1937.

Self-Help

Forgiveness

Luskin, F. *Forgive for Good.* San Francisco, CA: Harper Collins, 2001.

Priorities

Richardson, C. *Take Time for Your Life.* New York: Broadway Books, 1998.

RESOURCES

You can contact me through my website, www.art-of-getting-well.com, with questions or comments, to read the latest articles and self-care news, to have me speak to your group live or online, or to request consultation.

If you want to bring the Chronic Disease Self-Management Program to your facility, or to find out more about CDSMP, contact:

Stanford Patient Education Research Center
1000 Welch Rd., Ste. 204
Palo Alto CA 94304   (650) 723-7935
Website: www.stanford.edu/group/perc/

Or buy their book, *Living a Healthy Life with Chronic Conditions*, by Lorig, Holman, Sobel, Laurent, Gonzalez, and Munro (Bull Publishing, 1994). This is the original book on self-management, with an excellent section on exercise and two hundred helpful hints for making life easier.

All the references and resources listed below are available as of this writing in 2002. If you pick this up in 2013, I'm not guaranteeing anything. The list includes most of the books used in preparation of this book.

Alexander Technique

Stevens, C. *The Alexander Technique* (Charles Tuttle, 1987). The *British Medical Journal* calls this book an "excellent introduction."

Also contact the **Society of Teachers of the Alexander Technique (STAT)** at its website, www.stat.org.uk. This is a comprehensive site of Alexander-technique information, including a directory of practitioners covering the entire world.

Another good website is **www.alexandertechnique.com**.

Alternative Therapies

Cassileth, B. *The Alternative Medicine Handbook* (W.W. Norton, 1998). Describes and evaluates dozens of complementary and alternative approaches.

Anger Reduction

Donovan, F. *Dealing with Your Anger* (Hunter House, 2001).

Gentry, W.D. *Anger-Free: Ten Basic Steps to Managing Your Anger* (William Morrow, 1999).

Williams, R., and V. Williams. *Anger Kills: Seventeen Strategies for Controlling the Hostility That Can Harm Your Health* (Harper Perennial, 1994).

Assertiveness

Alberti, R., and M. Emmons. *Your Perfect Right: A Guide to Assertive Living,* 25th anniversary edition (Impact, 1995). This was one of the first self-help books, and it holds up very well.

Fensterheim, H., and J. Baer. *Don't Say Yes When You Want to Say No* (orig. pub. Dell, 1975; recently reissued).

Gordon, T. *Parent Effectiveness Training* (Peter H. Wyden, 1974).

Breathing

Cohen, D. *Arthritis: Stop Suffering and Start Moving* (Walker & Co., 1995). Includes many breathing exercises.

Ellis, G. *The Breath of Life: Mastering the Breathing Techniques of Pranayama and Qi Gong* (Newcastle, 1993). This contains mostly yoga breathing and postures. Beautiful pictures.

Centering Prayer

Keating, Fr. T. *Open Mind, Open Heart* (Harper Collins UK, 1994). Many consider this the best introduction to centering prayer.

Also check out the affiliated website, **www.centeringprayer.com**

☞ Chinese Medicine, Tai Chi, and Qi Gong

An excellent website is **www.acupuncture.com**. It contains referrals and information on all sorts of Chinese healing practices, current articles, and appropriate acupuncture points for different conditions. You can even sign up to send and receive e-mail there.

Gach, M.R. *Acupressure's Potent Points: A Guide to Self-Care for Common Ailments* (Bantam Doubleday Dell, 1990). Describes a useful self-care skill for many conditions, with some simple releases that can easily be learned for use with family members, friends, or patients.

Joiner, T.R. *Chinese Herbal Medicine Made Easy* (Hunter House, 2001).

Namikoshi, T. *The Complete Book of Shiatsu Therapy* (Japan Publishing, 1994). Shiatsu is probably the most widely used form of acupressure.

Williams, T., and H. Liping. *The Complete Illustrated Guide to Chinese Medicine: A Comprehensive System for Health and Fitness* (Thorsons, 1996).

⚊ *Tai Chi* ⚊

Chu, V. *Beginner's Tai Chi Chuan* (Unique, 2000).

Lam, P. *Tai Chi for Older Adults* (East Action Video, 1998). An excellent tape for beginners, nice and slow.

⚊ *Qi Gong* ⚊

Davis, D. *The Spirit of Qi Gong: Chinese Exercises for Longevity* (video, 1999). A beautiful video.

Wilson, S., and B. Kaplan. *Qi Gong for Beginners: Eight Easy Movements for Vibrant Health* (Sterling, 1997).

Many good **audiotapes** are also available describing qi gong breathing exercises and meditations.

Cognitive-Behavioral Psychology and Health

Beck, A. *Cognitive Therapy and the Emotional Disorders* (New American Library Trade, 1979 reprint edition). Actually, anything by Dr. Beck gives the basics of cognitive therapy in a very understandable way.

Ellis, A. *Reason and Emotion in Psychotherapy* (L. Stuart, 1962).

Coping with Chronic Illness

Feste, C. *The Physician Within* (Henry Holt and Company, 1993). An inspiring book by a truly inspiring person.

Lemaistre, J. *After the Diagnosis* (Ulysses, 1995).

Register, C. *Living with Chronic Illness* (Free Press, 1987). Reissued as *The Chronic Illness Experience*. Good advice on emotional coping and dealing with practical issues.

Royer, A. *Life with Chronic Illness* (Praeger, 1998 reissue).

Eating

Mellin, L. *The Solution* (Harper Perennial, 1998).

Roth, G. *Breaking Free of Compulsive Eating* (Plume, 1993).

Roth, G. *When Food Is Love* (Putnam, 1991).

Schwartz, B. *Diets Don't Work* (Breakthru, 1996).

Exercise

Hochschuler, S. and B. Reznik. *Treat Your Back Without Surgery* (Hunter House, 1998; second edition expected in 2002).

Torkelson, C. *Get Fit While You Sit* (Hunter House, 1999).

⌒ Feldenkrais

The Feldenkrais Guild of North America
3611 SW Hood Ave.
Portland OR 97201   (800) 775-2118
Website: www.feldenkrais.com

Includes books, tapes, and lists of practitioners around the world, even an online Feldenkrais lesson.

Meir Schneider's Center for Self-Healing
2218 48th Ave.
San Francisco CA 94116   (415) 665-9574
Website: www.self-healing.org

An offshoot of Feldenkrais that has had some amazing results, but there are few practitioners outside the Bay Area.

⌒ Financial and Legal Issues

Landay, D. *Be Prepared: The Complete Financial, Legal and Practical Guide to Living with Cancer, HIV, and Other Life-Challenging Conditions* (St. Martin's Press, 1998).

⌒ Forgiveness

Stanford Complementary Medicine Clinic (650) 498-5566

Luskin, F. *Forgive for Good* (Harper Collins San Francisco, 2001). Dr. Luskin also maintains a website: www.learningtoforgive.com.

⌒ Homeopathy

Cummings, S., and D. Ullman. *Everybody's Guide to Homeopathic Medicines: Safe and Effective Treatments for You and Your Family*, 3rd edition (JP Tarcher, 1997). By far the most popular American guide to homeopathic remedies.

National Center for Homeopathy
801 N. Fairfax St., Ste. 306
Alexandria VA 22314   (877) 624-0613
Website: www.homeopathic.org

Meditation and Awareness

www.meditationcenter.com

This is a wonderful resource! It includes many different meditations—all simple, all appropriate for beginners or veterans. Scores of other meditation-related websites also exist.

Benson, H. *The Relaxation Response* (Morrow, 1975).

Kabat-Zinn, J. *Wherever You Go, There You Are: Mindfulness Meditation in Everyday Life* (Hyperion, 1995).

Kabat-Zinn, J. *Full Catastrophe Living* (Delta, 1990).

Langer, E. *Mindfulness* (Perseus, 1990).

Mind/Body Connection

Here are some of my favorite books from among the vast number of books on the mind/body connection. They were used in researching this book and are seconded by the recommendations of people I trust.

Borysenko, J. *Minding the Body, Mending the Mind* (Addison-Wesley, 1987).

Martin, P. *The Healing Mind* (St. Martin's Press, 1997). This is one of the best.

Moyers, B. *Healing and the Mind* (Doubleday, 1993).

Ornstein, R., and D. Sobel. *The Healing Brain* (Simon and Schuster, 1987).

Ornstein, R., and D. Sobel. *Healthy Pleasures* (Addison Wesley, 1989).

Pert, C. *Molecules of Emotion* (Scribner, 1997).

Music and Rhythm Therapy

Clynes, M., and J. Walker. *Music, Mind and Brain* (Plenum Press, 1983).

Friedman, R.L. *The Healing Power of the Drum* (White Cliffs Media, 2000).

Organizing Your Time

Richardson, C. *Take Time for Your Life* (Broadway Books, 1999).

❧ Pain

www.darlenecohen.net
This website provides advice on and counseling for chronic pain.

Bresler, D. *Free Yourself from Pain* (Simon and Schuster, 1979). Getting control of pain through imagery and other self-help techniques.

Cohen, D. *Arthritis: Stop Suffering, Start Moving* (Walker and Company, 1995).

Cohen, D. *Finding a Joyful Life in the Heart of Pain* (Shambhala, 2000). Both of Cohen's books seamlessly weave the practical with the spiritual. *Arthritis* contains more specific exercises; *Joyful Life* teaches how to deal with the different kinds of pain life can bring.

Egoscue, P., and R. Gittines, *Pain-Free: A Revolutionary Method for Stopping Chronic Pain* (Bantam Doubleday, 2000). A movement program with shades of Feldenkrais.

Haylock, P.J., and C.P. Curtiss. *Cancer Doesn't Have to Hurt* (Hunter House, 1997).

Sarno, J. *The Mind/Body Prescription* (Warner Books, 1998). The psychological approach to dealing with chronic pain.

❧ Placebo Effect

Brody, H., and D. Brody. *The Placebo Response: How You Can Unleash the Body's Inner Pharmacy for Better Health* (Cliff Street Books, 2000).

❧ Recovery (Inspiring Stories)

Armstrong, L., with S. Jenkins. *It's Not About the Bike* (Putnam and Sons, 2000).

Barasch, M.I., and C. Hirshberg. *Remarkable Recovery* (Riverhead Books, 1995).

Cousins, N. *The Healing Heart* (W.W. Norton, 1983).

Cousins, N. *Anatomy of an Illness as Perceived by the Patient* (W.W. Norton, 1979).

LeShan, L. *Cancer as a Turning Point* (Dutton, 1989).

McCrum, R. *My Year Off* (W.W. Norton, 1998).

Schneider, M. *Self-healing: My Life and Vision* (Viking, 1989) The amazing story of Meir's healing himself from congenital blindness and his ongoing work healing others.

Siegel, B. *Love, Medicine and Miracles* (Harper & Row, 1986).

☞ Self-Esteem and Emotional Competence

Branden, N. *How to Raise Your Self-Esteem* (Bantam, 1987).

Branden, N. *Six Pillars of Self-Esteem* (Bantam, 1994).

Goleman, D. *Emotional Intelligence* (Bantam Books, 1995).

Persaud, R. *Staying Sane* (Metro, 1998).

Satir, V. *Self-Esteem* (Celestial Arts, 1975).

☞ Sex Information

Keesling, B. *Rx Sex: Making Love Is the Best Medicine* (Hunter House, 2000).

A website with lots of suggestions for sexual activities that don't involve inter-course is http://wso.williams.edu/peerh/sex/safesex/ssmenu.html. The intention is for safe sex, but much of it applies to low-energy or limited-mobility sex as well.

☞ Social Support

Lynch, J. *A Cry Unheard: New Insights into the Medical Consequences of Lone-liness* (Bancroft, 2000).

Lynch, J. *The Broken Heart: The Medical Consequences of Loneliness* (Basic Books, 1977).

Ornish, D. *Love and Survival* (Harper Perennial, 1998).

☞ Spiritual Dimensions of Health

Antonovsky, A. *Unraveling the Mystery of Health* (Jossey-Bass, 1987).

Bolen, J.S. *Close to the Bone* (Scribner, 1996).

Dossey, L. *Meaning and Medicine* (Bantam, 1992).

Remen, R.N. *The Human Patient* (Anchor Press, 1980).

Remen, R.N. *Kitchen Table Wisdom* (Riverhead Books, 1996).

☞ Visualization and Imagery

Assiogoli, R. *Psychosynthesis* (Hobbs Dorman, 1965). A psychological text on the theory behind IGI.

Naparstek, B. *The Health Journeys* series of guided-imagery tapes. Imagery individualized for most chronic and major problems. Order from: Image Paths Incorporated, 891 Moe Dr., Ste. C, Akron OH 44310-2538. Phone: (800) 800-8661. Website: www.healthjourneys.com

Rossman, M. *Healing Yourself*, six-tape set (Insight Publishing). Order from: PO Box 2070, Mill Valley CA 94942. Phone: (800) 726-2070, x03.

Rossman, M. *Guided Imagery for Self-Healing: An Essential Resource for Anyone Seeking Wellness* (New World Library, 2000).

Academy for Guided Imagery
(800) 726-2070
Website: www.interactiveimagery.com.

Trainings, books, tapes, and finding an imagery practitioner.

☞ Yoga

Devi, N. *The Healing Path of Yoga: Time-Honored Wisdom and Scientifically Proven Methods That Alleviate Stress, Open Your Heart and Enrich Your Life* (Three Rivers Press, 2000). All the yoga teachers I know seem to love this book.

Small, E. *Yoga with Eric Small: Adapted for Multiple Sclerosis and Other Disabilities* (video) (National Multiple Sclerosis Society, 1998). Available from the National Multiple Sclerosis Society of Southern California, (310) 749-4456.

Swami, S. *Integral Yoga Hatha* (Integral Yoga Distribution, 1998). A website affiliated with Swami Satchidananda is www.yogaville.org.

Walden, P. *Living Yoga* A.M./P.M.: *Yoga for Beginners* (video) (1998). Available at bookstores.

WOMEN LIVING WITH MULTIPLE SCLEROSIS

by Judith Lynn Nichols and Her Online Group of MS Sisters

Judith Lynn Nichols was diagnosed with multiple sclerosis in 1976. Puzzled by the differences between her experiences with the disease and the conventional medical response, she got on the Internet and eventually co-founded an online group of women dedicated to supporting each other in the fight against "the MonSter."

In this book, members of the group freely discuss intimate, emotional accounts of their experiences with MS. Some stories are painful, others are funny, often they are both. The range of topics includes family reactions to the MS diagnosis, workplace issues, sexuality and spirituality, depression and physical pain, loss of bladder and bowel control, and assistive devices and helpful tools. Read this book, and you will feel that someone *finally* understands.

288 pages ... Paperback $14.95

LIVING *BEYOND* MULTIPLE SCLEROSIS — A Women's Guide

by Judith Lynn Nichols and Her Online Group of MS Sisters; Foreword by Lily Jung, MD

They're back! The women whose frank, funny Internet chats became the basis for *Women Living with MS* return with a book that focuses on transcending the effects of MS. They discuss the elusive diagnosis, sustaining doctor/patient relationships, the latest treatments, tips for choosing and using assistive devices, and preparing Social Security disability applications. Time, energy, and sanity-saving techniques abound as the women share their pet peeves as well as the new talents, hobbies, and interests that have emerged since they have had to change their lives.

The book ends with moving commentary from the group about making peace with MS and finding ways to nourish their spirits, psyches, and imaginations for satisfying lives *beyond* MS.

288 pages ... Paperback $14.95

WHEN PARKINSON'S STRIKES EARLY: Voices, Choices, Resources and Treatment *by* Barbara Blake-Krebs, MA, and Linda Herman, MLS

An estimated 15 percent of all Parkinson's Disease (PD) sufferers are now diagnosed under the age of 50. The authors discuss the medical and social struggles faced by young people with Parkinson's and the support and resources available in the global PD community. They explain PD symptoms, the side effects of medications, and current surgery options, the benefits of patients developing a strong knowledge of their disease, and the unique impact early onset PD has on individuals and society.

The book is filled with the voices of young onset "Parkies" from around the world who refuse to forget their true worth or be forgotten. **All royalties from the sale of this book will be donated to Parkinson's Disease research.**

288 pages ... 4 illus. ... 19 b/w photos ... Paperback $15.95

To order go to www.hunterhouse.com *or call* 1-800-266-5592.
Free Media Mail shipping for all personal website orders

WOMEN LIVING WITH FIBROMYALGIA

by Mari Skelly ... Foreword *by* Devin Starlanyl

Using interviews, writings, discussions, and personal stories, this book deals with the real-life concerns of women with fibromyalgia (FM). Skelly highlights the strategies and therapies that a broad spectrum of women—from the single student pondering how FM will affect her as a woman, to the career professional exploring currently accepted treatments, to the mother trying to find energy to care for the family—use to face FM's many challenges. Topics include possible causes of the illness and why it especially affects women; fifty strategies for dealing with pain, fatigue, and sleep disturbances; and exploring spirituality in the face of a disease that is difficult to diagnose and for which there is no cure.

320 pages ... Paperback $16.95

ALTERNATIVE TREATMENTS FOR FIBROMYALGIA AND CHRONIC FATIGUE SYNDROME

by Mari Skelly ... Foreword *by* Paul Brown, MD, PhD

This guide combines interviews with professionals and the personal accounts of people living with FM and CFS. The stories offer a firsthand look at symptoms, treatments, and successes. They describe lifestyle adaptations and individualized medicine, diet, and activity regimens that can help other sufferers in their search for relief. The practitioner interviews cover acupuncture, tai chi, massage therapy, physical therapy, osteopathy, chiropractic, yoga, psychotherapy, energetic healing, and more, and include treatment plans and techniques to relieve symptoms.

320 pages ... Paperback $17.95 ... Second Edition

CHRONIC FATIGUE SYNDROME, FIBROMYALGIA & OTHER INVISIBLE ILLNESSES: The Comprehensive Guide

by Katrina Berne, PhD

Forewords *by* Robert M. Bennett, MD and Daniel L. Peterson, MD

This is a definitive guide to chronic fatigue syndrome (CFS) and fibromyalgia syndrome (FMS). Both illnesses are accompanied by a puzzling mix of physical, cognitive and emotional symptoms such as sore throat, headache, brain fog, sleep disturbance, balance problems, and depression. This book addresses what we know about causes of CFS and FMS, and whether they are related; the whole range of symptoms and diagnostic techniques; and proven and experimental treatment and self-care options. There is a chapter on CFS and FMS in children and invaluable advice on dealing with relationship issues and lifestyle changes. Similar conditions such as Gulf War Syndrome, lupus and post-polio syndrome are also discussed.

400 pages ... Paperback $17.95 ... Third Edition

POSITIVE OPTIONS FOR CROHN'S DISEASE by Joan Gomez, MD

Crohn's disease is an inflammatory bowel condition that, while nonfatal, can be devastating. This book discusses who is at risk and why, and addresses what can be done, including self-care.

192 pages ... 1 illus. ... Paperback $13.95

POSITIVE OPTIONS FOR LIVING WITH YOUR OSTOMY

by Dr. Craig A. White

This book is a complete, supportive guide to dealing with the practical and emotional aspects of life after ostomy surgery.

144 pages ... 4 illus. ... Paperback $12.95

POSITIVE OPTIONS FOR HIATUS HERNIA by Tom Smith, MD

A hiatus hernia is a common, potentially serious condition that occurs when the upper part of the stomach pushes through the diaphragm. This book describes tests, treatments, and self-help options.

128 pages ... 4 illus. ... 2 tables ... Paperback $12.95

POSITIVE OPTIONS FOR COLORECTAL CANCER by Carol Ann Larson

Colorectal cancer, the second leading cancer killer of adults in the U.S., is treatable if caught in time. This book tells you everything you need to know about prevention, diagnosis, and treatment.

168 pages ... 10 illus. ... Paperback $12.95

POSITIVE OPTIONS FOR REFLEX SYMPATHETIC DYSTROPHY (RSD)

by Elena Juris

RSD, also called Complex Regional Pain Syndrome, is characterized by severe nerve pain and extreme sensitivity to touch. This book covers medical information, practical advice, and holistic therapies.

224 pages ... 2 illus. ... Paperback $14.95

POSITIVE OPTIONS FOR ANTIPHOSPHOLIPID SYNDROME (APS)

by Triona Holden

Also called Hughes syndrome and "sticky blood," APS is implicated in many serious health problems. This book identifies the symptoms and provides important information on diagnosis and treatment.

144 pages ... Paperback $12.95

POSITIVE OPTIONS FOR SEASONAL AFFECTIVE DISORDER (SAD)

by Fiona Marshall and Peter Cheevers

About 10 million Americans suffer from SAD. This book helps distinguish the condition from classic depression and chronic fatigue, and suggests ways to alleviate the symptoms and live optimally.

144 pages ... Paperback $12.95

POSITIVE OPTIONS FOR POLYCYSTIC OVARY SYNDROME (PCOS)

by Christine Craggs-Hinton and Adam Balen, MD

> PCOS is a leading cause of infertility and affects 5–10 percent of women of childbearing age. This book covers symptoms; diagnosis and medical treatments; active self-help; and complementary therapies, including exercise, the use of herbs, and lifestyle changes.

168 pages ... 17 illus. ... Paperback $12.95

POSITIVE OPTIONS FOR CHILDREN WITH ASTHMA by O.P. Jaggi, MD

> This manual helps parents better understand and cope with the frightening disease of asthma, and offers advice on creating an allergen-free environment, recognizing warning signs, and the various diagnostic procedures and treatment options available.

168 pages ... 38 illus. ... Paperback $12.95

ANEMIA IN WOMEN by Joan Gomez, MD

> Undiagnosed anemia in women can lead to infertility, premature delivery, fainting, and mental confusion. Joan Gomez discusses why women develop anemia more than men, the two main types of anemia, their treatment, and self-help options.

176 pages ... Paperback $12.95

THYROID PROBLEMS IN WOMEN AND CHILDREN by Joan Gomez, MD

> This book helps readers understand the health impact of thyroid disorders and the many treatment options. Special chapters cover pregnant women, infants and children, adolescents, and women over 50. Also discusses vitamins, the role of iodine, and the role of stress.

208 pages ... Paperback $14.95

THE IBS HEALING PLAN: Natural Ways to Beat Your Symptoms

by Theresa Cheung

> Information and help for those suffering from the abdominal pain, bloating, and irregular bowel habits that are the symptoms of IBS. The plan focuses on five key areas: diet, supplements, complementary therapies, stress management, and working with your doctor.

168 pages ... 9 illus. ... Paperback $14.95

SELF-HELP FOR HYPERVENTILATION SYNDROME: Recognizing and Correcting Your Breathing-Pattern Disorder by Dinah Bradley

> Chronic hyperventilation symptoms include breathlessness, chest pain, palpitations, broken sleep, stomach problems, dizziness, and anxiety. This book explains causes and symptoms and presents a well-tested program that will help readers to breathe freely again.

128 pages ... 30 illus. ... 3rd Edition ... Paperback $13.95

To order go to www.hunterhouse.com *or call* 1-800-266-5592.
Free Media Mail shipping for all personal website orders